CLINICAL HANDBOOK OF NEONATAL PAIN MANAGEMENT FOR NURSES

Tara Marko, MSN, RNC-NIC, is an adjunct professor of maternal–child nursing at California State University, San Marcos (CSUSM), and a staff nurse at Rady Children's Hospital San Diego. She is also a faculty advisor with the CSUSM chapter of Sigma Theta Tau International Nursing Honor Society. She received her diploma from Bayonne Medical Center School of Nursing, her bachelor of science in nursing from New Jersey City University, and her master of science in nursing from Seton Hall University.

Michelle L. Dickerson, MSN-Ed, RNC-NIC, RN-BC, is a nurse and nurse educator. She has worked in neonatal intensive care as a bedside nurse and as an educator for 17 years, striving to provide the most compassionate and sensitive care possible to fragile and compromised newborns. An advocate for mitigating pain in neonates, she has championed initiatives to improve the identification and management of neonatal pain through example and education in her current workplace. Ms. Dickerson is currently a neonatal intensive care unit (NICU) educator in a Level III neonatal intensive care unit, where she engages in efforts to bring awareness to and management of neonatal pain.

Ms. Dickerson received her master's in nursing education from the University of Phoenix and is currently on the last leg of a long journey toward achieving her PhD in nursing education. She is a neonatal resuscitation program instructor; a sugar, temperature, airway, blood pressure, labs, and emotional support (STABLE) instructor; a certified breast feeding counselor; and is nationally certified as a high-risk neonatal intensive care nurse. She has been recognized by her peers through nomination of nursing excellence awards citing a commitment and passion to the continuing education and promotion of patient care. Ms. Dickerson hopes to promote the knowledge and expertise she has gained through years of nursing to future generations of nurses through her academic commitments.

CLINICAL HANDBOOK OF NEONATAL PAIN MANAGEMENT FOR NURSES

Tara Marko, MSN, RNC-NIC

Michelle L. Dickerson, MSN-Ed, RNC-NIC, RN-BC

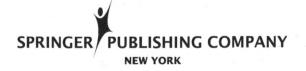

SPRINGER PUBLISHING COMPANY
NEW YORK

Springer Publishing Company, LLC
11 West 42nd Street
New York, NY 10036
www.springerpub.com

Acquisitions Editor: Elizabeth Nieginski
Composition: diacriTech

ISBN: 978-0-8261-9437-4
e-book ISBN: 978-0-8261-9438-1

16 17 18 / 5 4 3 2 1

The author and the publisher of this Work have made every effort to use sources believed to be reliable to provide information that is accurate and compatible with the standards generally accepted at the time of publication. Because medical science is continually advancing, our knowledge base continues to expand. Therefore, as new information becomes available, changes in procedures become necessary. We recommend that the reader always consult current research and specific institutional policies before performing any clinical procedure. The author and publisher shall not be liable for any special, consequential, or exemplary damages resulting, in whole or in part, from the readers' use of, or reliance on, the information contained in this book. The publisher has no responsibility for the persistence or accuracy of URLs for external or third-party Internet websites referred to in this publication and does not guarantee that any content on such websites is, or will remain, accurate or appropriate.

Library of Congress Cataloging-in-Publication Data
Names: Marko, Tara, author. | Dickerson, Michelle, L. author.
Title: Clinical handbook of neonatal pain management for nurses / Tara Marko,
    Michelle L. Dickerson.
Description: New York, NY : Springer Publishing Company, LLC, [2017] |
    Includes bibliographical references and index.
Identifiers: LCCN 2016020118| ISBN 9780826194374 | ISBN 9780826194381 (e-book)
Subjects: | MESH: Pain Management—nursing | Infant, Newborn | Neonatal
    Nursing—methods | Pain—drug therapy
Classification: LCC RJ365 | NLM WY 157.3 | DDC 618.92/0472—dc23 LC record available
at https://lccn.loc.gov/2016020118

Special discounts on bulk quantities of our books are available to corporations, professional associations, pharmaceutical companies, health care organizations, and other qualifying groups. If you are interested in a custom book, including chapters from more than one of our titles, we can provide that service as well.
For details, please contact:
Special Sales Department, Springer Publishing Company, LLC
11 West 42nd Street, 15th Floor, New York, NY 10036-8002
Phone: 877-687-7476 or 212-431-4370; Fax: 212-941-7842
E-mail: sales@springerpub.com

Printed in the United States of America by McNaughton & Gunn.

To my husband, Scott, and my two boys, who are my biggest support and inspiration.
I love you so much.

—Tara Marko

I dedicate this book in memory of Paige, for all she has taught me.
—Michelle L. Dickerson

Contents

Section IV: Integration of Treatment Methods

Section V: Special Populations

Foreword

As a neonatologist, I have grown to understand the importance
of identifying and managing neonatal pain and the detrimental
effects of not doing so. Pain management in the neonate is a subject that has been misunderstood for many years. The prevention
of pain in neonates should be the goal of all caregivers, because
repeated painful exposures have the potential for deleterious
consequences in both the short and long term. We are just beginning to understand pain perception and management in the neonate and I believe this book provides a great tool to help the
practitioner understand and reach that very worthy goal.

The content of this book will help any neonatal clinician gain
a deeper understanding of the physiology of neonatal pain, as
well as pharmaceutical and nonpharmaceutical pain management methods. Over the years, neonatal medicine has been subject to the unfortunate misconception that neonates do not feel
pain as acutely as do adults and, as a result, neonatal pain management and its long-term sequelae have long been underserved
and undermanaged. The difficulty associated with accurately
and comprehensively assessing pain by health care providers
has contributed to the many challenges related to effective neonatal pain management. Much progress has been made in recent
years to bridge the gap between understanding how neonates
process pain, how neonates display pain, and interventions for
mitigating neonatal pain, from very premature infants to term
infants suffering withdrawal. This handbook provides a tool for
nursing and health care workers responsible for neonatal care to
help bridge those gaps.

The introductory chapters provide detailed information about the physiology of pain—a topic that has not always been a focus in neonatal care education and provides a foundation for that understanding. Detailed explanation of the pharmacological and nonpharmacological approaches to pain management provides a neonatal clinician with a deeper understanding of the properties of available medications and the neonatal response. Discussion of the role of the family and the special care considerations associated with the premature infant provides guidance for the integration of a variety of treatment approaches to serve the neonatal population. Especially helpful is the end-of-life and palliative care discussion, a much debated topic of pain and pain management in neonatal nursing and medicine. The chapters addressing developmental care approaches and the interdisciplinary team approach to managing pain are especially thoughtful and applicable to any care setting. Neonatal nurses face many challenges in their role as advocates in protecting their fragile patients and this book provides a resource for meeting those obligations as part of the health care team.

The collaborative efforts of Tara Marko and Michelle L. Dickerson have resulted in an eminently useful clinical reference product that all neonatal clinicians can use as a reliable resource in addressing the varied and significant pain management needs of their vulnerable patients.

John Tadros, MD, FAAP
Co-Chief of Neonatology
RWJBarnabas Health
Jersey City Medical Center
Jersey City, New Jersey

Preface

The *Clinical Handbook of Neonatal Pain Management for Nurses* represents a work of passion and love on a topic that is very timely and important. Increasingly, we realize the effects of pain and the need to protect our most fragile patients. We wrote this book after recognizing the need for a text that emphasized pain management and to start an in-depth, multidisciplinary conversation about neonatal pain. With this book, we hope to bring awareness and understanding of neonatal pain to those already committed to the smallest patients and those interested in joining the specialty.

The book is a collection of information about how pain works, how pain affects neonates physiologically and developmentally, and how to assess and treat pain in various ways. What sets this book apart from much of the information available is the comprehensive nature of the information and the balance between appropriate pharmacological measures and nonpharmacological, holistic interventions. Our aim is to make the text clear, concise, and to provide valuable information to the entire health care team. Neonatal pain management is the responsibility of everyone on the team—physicians, nurse practitioners, nurses, pharmacists, respiratory therapists, speech/occupational/physical therapists, and family members—to ensure that the needs of neonates are met and to advocate for our most fragile patients.

The book also addresses special circumstances, such as prematurity, neonatal abstinence syndrome, and end-of-life care, as well as basic and useful information to care for all neonates who may experience pain. Chapters 9 and 10 provide unique perspectives and information that focus on a multidisciplinary approach to understanding and managing neonatal pain. Chapter 9 provides examples and case studies that promote communication techniques within the health care team to manage neonatal pain. Chapter 12 focuses on the premature infant and the unique challenges the compromised premature infant poses in recognizing and treating pain. Finally, Chapter 14 addresses the difficult topic of end-of-life challenges and palliative care. This chapter provides suggestions and thoughts on how best to address decision making and pain management to promote a peaceful, dignified death.

We are honored to contribute to this important conversation.

Tara Marko
Michelle L. Dickerson

Expert Reviewer

Michele Beaulieu, DNP, ARNP, NNP-BC, is a full-time neonatal nurse practitioner as well as an author, researcher, and educator. She earned her doctor of nursing (DNP) degree from Case Western Reserve University Frances Payne Bolton School of Nursing. In addition to her full-time neonatal practice, she has been the column editor for "Pointers in Practical Pharmacology" in *Neonatal Network: The Journal of Neonatal Nursing*, author and reviewer of various peer-reviewed manuscripts and books, and is co-investigator for several research studies. Her research interests include perinatal safety, extremely low-birth-weight infants, neonatal abstinence syndrome, and the management of high-risk newborns in the delivery room. She has developed and taught clinical and online courses for undergraduate and graduate nursing programs. She is a member of Sigma Theta Tau (Delta Beta Chapter) and is actively involved in several neonatal and women's health professional organizations, among them the Florida Association of Neonatal Nurse Practitioners (FANNP).

Acknowledgments

First, I want to acknowledge the dedicated team that helped bring this book together: Michelle L. Dickerson, my colleague and friend who has taught me so much about neonatal nursing and pain management; Dr. Michele Beaulieu, who lent her expertise in reviewing this book; Dr. John Tadros, for his wonderful words, encouragement, and personal commitment to our special population; Elizabeth Nieginski, for noticing the importance of this issue and bringing Michelle and me on board to author this work and facilitating all of the logistics; Rachel Landes, for assisting and guiding us throughout the process; and the entire production team at Springer Publishing Company, for making this dream a reality.

Also, I'd like to thank my colleagues at Jersey City Medical Center for mentoring me when I was a new nurse and then becoming my wonderful friends and colleagues. The nurses at Rady Children's Hospital are experts in neonatal care and have taught me so much. I acknowledge the nurses at Tri-City Medical Center, who are committed to expert practice, especially in pain management. I thank the dedicated and wonderful professors at New Jersey City University and California State University, San Marcos, who are experts in their field. And my students, who keep me on my toes and share their beautiful enthusiasm with me.

And to the patients and families I care for: I am forever grateful to be a part of your life and to be able to help you through this difficult time.

Tara Marko

First, I would like to thank Tara for asking me to be a part of this labor of love in creating this amazing book—I was and am honored to be a partner on this journey! Many, many thanks to Elizabeth Nieginski for her faith in two nurses and believing they could create such a necessary contribution and providing the resources to do so; more thanks to Rachel Landes for her never-ending patience with endless questions and her support throughout this amazing journey; and special thanks to Dr. Michele Beaulieu for her comprehensive and constructive feedback, which truly helped make this book relevant and current.

I would like to express gratitude to my colleagues and peers who provided support, encouragement, and cheered me on through the entire process . . . your support and unfailing faith are forever appreciated.

I would like to thank my family for their unending support, their necessary patience, for tolerating my indifference and absences, and for never disturbing my piles of papers during the course of writing this book—you have always been my source of inspiration to do better and do more, none of which I could ever achieve without you.

Michelle L. Dickerson

Neonatal Pain

History and Overview of Neonatal Pain

The study of pain in neonates is relatively new and still evolving. Before the 1980s, pain in the neonate was disputed and often dismissed. The idea that neonates do not experience pain is not new. Charles Darwin, in his famous work *The Expression of the Emotions in Man and Animals*, wrote that even though newborns exhibit pain reactions, these were only reflexive and babies were incapable of experiencing and expressing true pain (Darwin, 1872). Darwin's belief, coupled with research by scientists such as Dr. Flechsig, who equated the absence of myelination in some of the baby's nervous system as the system's inability to function (Cope, 1998). This idea was so widely believed that even operations, including open-heart surgery, were carried out without the use of analgesics or anesthetics (Cope, 1998). It was thought that neonatal nervous systems were so immature that they did not feel pain and that lack of myelination translated into a decreased or disorganized response to pain. It is now known that incomplete myelination only leads to a slower conduction of pain, not an absence of pain. This decreased speed is offset, however, by the shorter distance the impulse needs to travel to reach the neonatal brain. Myelination is usually complete by the second to third trimester. There was a belief that because the infant would not remember the pain, it was not necessary to provide relief from pain. Another common concern was that the risks of pain relief exceeded the benefits when it came to pharmacologic and anesthetic use. Today, it is understood that pain is detrimental to term and preterm infants and that these patients have a worse pain experience than an adult or older child. This realization began with a landmark paper published by Anand and Hickey in 1987, which was one of the first peer-reviewed trials to study pain in the neonatal population. In this article, it was made clear that even a fetus is capable of experiencing pain and urged clinicians to humanely treat pain in this population as adults and older children would be treated (Anand & Hickey, 1987). In 1987, the American Academy of Pediatrics (AAP) released a statement on neonatal pain control with consensus from three of their committees: the Committee on Fetus and Newborn and the Committee on Drugs, the Section on Anesthesiology and the Section on Surgery. The statement confirmed that there are now ways to safely use anesthesia and analgesia for surgical procedures and such treatment should be given by following the guidelines for any high-risk patient (AAP, 1987). Practice still needed time to catch up though. In 1997, a study was published on neonatal intensive care units (NICUs), which found that 2,134 invasive procedures were performed in 1 week on 239 patients and only 0.8% of these patients received analgesics (Johnson, Collinge, & Henderson, 1997). Then, in 2001, the AAP Committee on Psychosocial Aspects of Children and Family Health, along with the American Pain Society (APS) Task Force on Pain in Infants, Children, and Adolescents, published a call-to-action statement for the treatment of pediatric pain. In this statement, they directly addressed the critical need for pain management with all types of pediatric pain (acute injuries, chronic pain, procedures, surgery, etc.), and some of the barriers keeping patients from receiving the pain control that they deserve (American Academy of Pediatrics, 2001). A few years later a study was published that demonstrated about one third of the study neonates received analgesia for painful procedures (Simons et al., 2003).

Two studies have addressed whether infants can process noxious stimulation at the cortical level. Using real-time, near-infrared spectroscopy to detect changes in cortical blood flow, both studies showed that noxious stimuli activated the primary somatosensory cortex in newborns (Bartocci, Bergqvist, Lagercrantz, & Anand, 2006; Slater et al., 2006). This was shown to occur in even preterm infants, the youngest of whom were tested at 25 weeks gestational age (Slater et al., 2006).

The current movement is toward pain prevention and treatment, rather than treatment alone. Because of the adverse effects stress can have on the developing neonate, eliminating or minimizing as much stress as possible has become standard practice. Standardized policies and procedures regarding pain management have been put into place in many organizations.

Pain assessment and management are one of the most important components of patient care. Pain is often referred to as the "fifth vital sign" (a phrase introduced by The Joint Commission), along with heart rate, respiration, blood pressure, and temperature, because of the powerful indicator pain is of the patient's current condition.

Pain is a complex topic that is especially difficult to conceptualize in the neonatal population. Practitioners for adult patients typically base treatment on verbal descriptions regarding pain level and tolerance, yet neonates do not yet have the capacity to relay this information. This leads to a high risk of misinterpreted pain responses and inadequate pain relief in this fragile population, who, unfortunately, are most affected by pain. Neonates sometimes offer physiologic cues to signal pain, but this may be masked or confused with concurrent conditions and comorbidities. For this reason, pain should be at the forefront of all clinical practice and pain relief should be administered if any pain signs are noticed or anticipated.

DEFINING PAIN

There are many ways to describe pain. The International Association for the Study of Pain (IASP) definition of *pain* as, "an unpleasant sensory and emotional experience associated with actual or potential tissue damage, or described in terms of such damage" is derived from a 1964 definition by Harold Merskey (1979, p. 250). If the patient is an adult and a good historian, simply asking him or her to describe the pain, its location, quality, duration, exacerbating and relieving factors, whether there has been previous injury and any other associating symptoms (such as swelling, numbness, erythema, etc.) will give clues as to what is causing the pain and how relief can be provided. But neonates, unlike adults or even older children, are not able to verbalize such sensations. Neonates also give nonspecific and inconsistent cues that may become masked in their underlying pathology (such as a premature infant having an apneic episode in which pain may not be considered as part of the problem). When treating this population, care providers have to be attuned to often subtle or complicated symptoms. In some cases, providers should treat based on the fact that they are performing an invasive procedure known to cause pain. Inability to express pain in a traditional manner in no way negates the fact that pain is being experienced.

ANATOMY AND PAIN PATHWAYS

DEVELOPMENT

Responses to somatic stimuli begin at an early age. Reflex responses to stimuli begin around 7.5 weeks postconception in the perioral skin and continue to develop in the palms of the hands before finally reaching the limbs by about 13 to 14 weeks. Peripheral pain receptors are in place systemically by around 20 weeks postconception (Stevens, 1999). By 21 weeks, there is dendritic arborization. At around 22 weeks postconception, nerve tracts in the spinal cord to the brain stem and connections with the thalamocortical fibers are in place. But it is not until 32 weeks that the descending, inhibitory fibers are complete. These fibers aid in blunting full pain response and experience. Therefore, a lack of neurotransmitters in the descending tract suggests a lack of complete neuromodulating mechanisms in the preterm infant, making the infant more sensitive to pain than older children and adults (Anand et al., 2006).

Nociception is the most common pain pathway. Nociceptors are sensory receptors that are located throughout the body and are activated by physical, chemical, or heat stimuli. First, painful sensory stimuli are introduced; these can be actual tissue damage, muscle spasms, or even anticipated tissue damage.

Most pain originates from damage to body tissues. A stimulus is introduced, perceived by the nociceptors, then sent through the spinal cord and into the brain for interpretation. A stimulus is transmitted first through tiny afferent nerve fibers in the spinal cord. The fibers that are most responsible for pain are the afferent A-delta and C-fibers (Adriaensen, Gybels, Handwerker, & Van Hees, 1983). These fibers are the first-order neurons and they begin the pain-perception process. A-delta fibers are found primarily in the skin and muscle, and C-fibers are found in muscle, periosteum, and visceral organs. A-delta fibers are myelinated fibers that produce rapid sharp, pricking, and piercing sensations. This pain is usually localized. In contrast, C-fibers are unmyelinated (or poorly so), and conduct temperature, chemical, or strong physical signals. Pain elicited from the C-fibers is a dull, aching, or burning pain that is more diffuse. Of note, there are other fibers responsible for sensation related to pain, such as A-alpha and A-beta fibers. A-alpha and A-beta fibers transmit nonpainful sensations such as pressure, soft touch, and vibration. These nonpainful sensations can be either beneficial or detrimental to pain management by either contributing to stimulation overload or by helping to block painful messages.

The stimuli then travel through to the spinal cord, to the dorsal root ganglia, through to the dorsal horn, and up to the thalamus. This begins the involvement of the second-order neurons. The tract from the dorsal horn to the thalamus is called the spinothalamic tract and it is divided into two pathways: the lateral pathway called the neospinothalamic (NST) tract and the medial pathway called the paleospinothalamic (PST) tract. The NST tract transmits pain directly to the sensory cortex, where it is interpreted. The PST tract synapses in other parts of the brain, such as the limbic system and the reticular formation, which are areas of the brain responsible for emotion and circadian rhythm. A-beta fibers make synapses in the spinal dorsal horn close to synapses of the A-delta and C-fibers. This dorsal horn connection means that input from touch fibers can enter the spinal cord and synapse or communicate with cells carrying nociceptive input. This is an important reason that techniques, such as massage, light touch, acupuncture/acupressure, and other alternative measures, work to aid in pain management.

Pain stimuli may be influenced by neuroregulators. Neuroregulators are chemicals that inhibit, enable, or even enhance painful stimuli. There are two types: neurotransmitters and neuromodulators. Neurotransmitters, such as epinephrine, norepinephrine, acetylcholine, and dopamine, work to either slow or accelerate postsynaptic nerve activity. Neuromodulators are endogenous opiates and help in pain relief. They consist of large amino acid peptides, such as alpha-endorphins, beta-endorphins, and enkephalins, which act similarly to morphine with increased potency. Endorphins are produced in the anterior pituitary gland and hypothalamus. They are larger peptides and longer acting than enkephalins. Enkephalins are more diffuse throughout the brain and dorsal horn. Several types of endorphins and enkephalins have been identified and each acts on a highly specific opiate receptor in the central nervous system (CNS).

Once the pain signal reaches the brain, it is processed at three levels: the thalamus, midbrain, and cortex. These areas work together to interpret and respond to stimuli. The thalamus relays sensory data from the NST and PST tracts. The midbrain alerts the cortex to be aware of incoming stimuli. Lastly, the cortex discriminates and interprets the stimuli. This demonstrates that the painful stimuli must pass through many areas of the brain, which sometimes includes behavioral and emotional centers. All of this happens in a matter of seconds (Figure 1.1).

Almost all painful stimuli cause some degree of tissue damage (e.g., heel lancing, venipuncture, catheterization, difficult adhesive tape removal). This damage leads to a release of chemicals, such as noradrenaline, bradykinin, histamine, prostaglandins, purines, cytokines, 5-HT, leukotrienes, nerve growth factor, and neuropeptides, which sensitize the receptors. This sensitization occurs to make sure the body is aware of the painful stimuli and can act to stop the stimuli and begin repair. These chemicals can also lead to a decrease in the nociception threshold, ectopic discharges, and accumulation of sodium (Na) channels, especially with repeated exposure to pain (Devor, 1994).

Pain is processed in four main ways: transduction, transmission, modulation, and perception (Box 1.1).

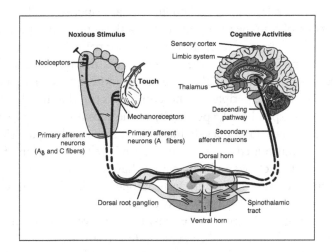

FIGURE 1.1. Noceptive stimulus received at the periphery → travels through the dorsal horn of the spinal cord to the dorsal root ganglia → thalamus → through the spinothalamic tracts (paleospinothalamic [PST] and neospinothalamic [NST]) → NST goes to the sensory cortex → PST goes to limbic system and reticular formation.

BOX 1.1 Processing Pain
Transduction—When nociceptors are exposed to a noxious stimulus *Transmission*—Path of the stimulus sent from the site of transduction to the dorsal horn of the spinal cord, then to the brain stem, finally to higher levels of the brain *Modulation*—Painful stimuli may be inhibited or enhanced by neurotransmitters on the way to perception *Perception*—Pain signals reach their final destination in the brain and are interpreted

PAIN THEORIES

Most information known about pain is related to the adult pain experience. One prominent pain theory is the gate control theory introduced in 1965 by Melzack and Wall. This theory explores the fact that pain is more than just a physiologic response; other variables, such as behavioral and emotional responses, influence perception of pain. Because neonates lack the context to apply the stimuli, this gate is more likely to be open for painful messages to reach the brain. Let us further describe this theory. The gating process occurs in the spinal cord. A-delta and C-fibers send pain impulses from the periphery. These impulses travel to the dorsal horns of the spinal cord, specifically to the substantia gelatinesa. The cells of the substantia gelatinesa either stop or allow pain signals to be transmitted to the T-cells. When T-cell activity is inhibited, the gate is closed and pain signals have a reduced chance of reaching the brain. When the gate is open, pain signals travel directly to the brain (Melzack & Wall, 1965).

Similar "gating" mechanisms exist in the nerve fiber descending from the thalamus and cerebral cortex. These are the areas of the brain that control thoughts and emotions. When pain occurs, a person's thoughts and emotions can modify the perception of pain. Neonates, unfortunately, lack language abilities, life experience, and control over thoughts and emotions to assist in this gating process. Neonates benefit from comfort measures that help to reduce pain by reducing agitation, promoting sleep, and decreasing a feeling of disorganization (AAP and Canadian Paediatric Society, 2006). Other theories have been proposed against the gate control theory, some arguing a more dynamic and less linear path of pain interpretation.

Another theory related to pain that has significant bearing on the neonate is the theory of wind-up. Wind-up is a phenomenon in which repeated exposure to the same noxious stimulus leads to an exaggerated response and this response continues even after the noxious stimulus is withdrawn (McMahon, Koltzenburg, Tracey, & Turk, 2013). With repeated moderate to severe pain, N-methyl-L-D-aspartate (NMDA) receptors are activated, which produces a wind-up effect, changing intracellular calcium ion concentrations and creating synaptic buildup of excitatory amino acids. Pain intensity, duration, and surface distribution become greater than expected for a particular stimulus (Coderre, Katz, Vaccarino, & Melzack, 1993).

TYPES OF PAIN (NOCICEPTIVE, NEUROPATHIC, SOMATIC, VISCERAL, ACUTE, CHRONIC)

One of the ways to describe pain is from its source. Pain can originate from several different locations and manifest in many different ways. Nociceptive pain is perceived by afferent nerve fibers (as described in Figure 1.1). This refers to a stimulus activating the nociceptors in body tissue, and then traveling through the spinal cord and brain for interpretation and action. Nociceptors are so named because of their affinity to transmit noxious stimuli (Sherrington, 1906). They perceive all potential risks to body tissues, including thermal, mechanical, and chemical risks. Neuropathic pain is perceived by deafferent nerve fibers. The IASP defines *neuropathic pain* as "pain caused by a lesion or disease of the somatosensory system" (Merskey, Lindblom, Mumford, Nathan, & Sunderland, 1994). This is basically pain not caused by a painful stimulus, but by a dysfunction or defect in the neurological system resulting in pain. This is rare in neonates, but may occur with traumatic brain injury from delivery, meningitis, or some other encephalopathic condition.

Pain can also be described as somatic or visceral. Somatic pain affects the skin, bone, muscle, blood vessels, and connective tissue. Visceral pain affects the vital organs and the linings of body cavities. An example of somatic pain would be a venipuncture. An example of visceral pain would be insertion of a chest or gastrointestinal tube.

Acute pain is temporary pain that is expected to last no longer than 6 months. Examples of this would be procedural pain or pain from an acute injury. Chronic pain is pain that lasts or is expected to last longer than 6 months. Chronic pain is rare in neonates. Examples of chronic pain would be pain from incurable neurodegenerative diseases or cancer. In the APS's latest statement they indicate the significance of chronic pain in the pediatric population and stress the importance of improving patient functioning and quality of life. The APS also recommends the use of psychological interventions, such as relaxation techniques and parent interventions, for all children with chronic pain.

PHYSIOLOGIC, BEHAVIORAL, AND BIOCHEMICAL RESPONSES TO PAIN

When adults experience acute pain, they exhibit a sympathetic nervous system response that can be observed as an increase in heart rate, blood pressure, respiration, anxiety, hormonal fluctuation, and inflammation. Various studies have found that neonates and preterm infants exhibit similar physiologic responses to pain (Table 1.1).

TABLE 1.1 Effects of Pain
Physiologic Response
Heart rate increase or fluctuation
Blood pressure increase or fluctuation
Increased PO_2 (partial pressure of oxygen), SaO_2 (oxygen saturation; initially)
Decreased PO_2, SaO_2 (prolonged stress)
Increased work of breathing
Apnea
Hypercapnea
V/Q mismatch
Increase in intracranial pressure
Vomiting
Diarrhea, which may result in diaper rash

(continued)

TABLE 1.1 Effects of Pain (*continued*)

Diaphoresis

Dilated pupils

Slow weight gain, weight loss, failure to thrive

Ileus

Urinary retention

Behavioral Response

Intense or high-pitched cry

Difficult to console

Constant need to be consoled

Frowning, grimacing, brow furrow

Eye closure or aversion

Disorganized or frantic body movements

Increased tone

Decreased activity, "shutting down" (prolonged stress)

Tremors

Hyperalert state

Erratic sleep pattern

Feeding difficulties or increased feeds, which may result in vomiting

Behavioral Response

Increased plasma renin activity

Increased epinephrine and norepinephrine

Increased cortisol levels

Increased glucose

Increased lactate

Increased pyruvate

Release in growth hormones, aldosterone, and glucagon

Sodium or water retention

(*continued*)

TABLE 1.1 Effects of Pain (*continued*)
Protein catabolism
Decreased immune function
Decreased insulin
Decreased prolactin
Decreased platelet adhesion/hypercoagulability
Long-Term Response
Increased length of stay in the hospital
Higher mortality
Increased sensitivity to pain

Sources: Anand (1990); Anand (1993); Anand and Hickey (1987); Burddeau and Kleiber (1991); Gardner, Carter, Enzman-Hines, and Hernandez (2011); and Hall and Anand (2005).

Tissue damage results in a cascade of events that lead to hyperalgesia or enhanced pain in response to all stimuli, as well as sensitization of nocicepetors at and around the injured area. Hyperalgesia and sensitization occur with most somatic and visceral injuries. For example, in the presence of pharyngitis, mere swallowing is painful (McMahon et al., 2013).

A noxious stimulus leads to action in the nociceptive fibers that propagates not only to the CNS, but also into surrounding areas. There is a release of neuropeptides, such as substance P, calcitonin gene-related peptide (CGRP), and neurokinin A (NKA). These substances can stimulate epidermal cells and immune cells or lead to vasodilation, plasma extravasation, and smooth muscle contraction, which can lead to surrounding areas becoming inflamed, erythemic, and tense (McMahon et al., 2013).

The preterm infant is especially susceptible to negative effects of pain. The preterm infant experiences increased stress and activity in the nociceptive pathways after prolonged periods of exposure to painful stimuli. After repeated painful experiences, the preterm infant exhibits pain responses when exposed to other routine caregiving activities (e.g., suctioning, repositioning, and diaper changes; Evans, Vogelpohl, Bourguignon, & Morcott, 1997), further illustrating the wind-up theory. A neonate or preterm neonate also begins to develop associations between an action and the painful stimulus. For example, the neonate will elicit a pain response and may cry out or fight when an alcohol wipe is brushed across his heel. The neonate is expecting the painful prick of a lancet to follow. If exposure is especially prolonged or traumatic, aversions may develop. For example, a preterm infant may reject a bottle or the breast because of repeated and prolonged endotracheal intubation. Even with developmentally appropriate care, true oral aversions may take months or even years to correct and a gastrointestinal tube may need to be surgically place until the oral aversion resolves.

Neonates may have a higher pain threshold in the upper extremities than in the lower extremities, leading to increased sensitivity to pain in the lower extremities. The descending inhibitory fibers grow from the supraspinal brainstem nuclei, only reaching the cervical section of the spinal cord by 30 to 32 weeks; they have not reached the lumbar spine by 30 weeks, which allows for an increased sensitivity for pain in the lower extremities (Anand, 2007). This is an important factor to consider from a clinical standpoint when there is choice as to which procedure to perform such as deciding between an intravenous catheter site and a heel stick for blood draw.

REGULATIONS/PROFESSIONAL GUIDELINES

As the discussion and study of pain for all patients grows, many governmental, regulatory, and professional organizations have issue and rules and guidelines regarding pain management. Beginning in 2001, California, for example, mandated that health care professionals document pain assessment whenever they documented vital signs.

According to the National Association of Neonatal Nurses (NANN; 2008) guidelines:

1. Education and competency validation in pain assessment and management shall be conducted during orientation and at regularly defined intervals throughout employment for all nurses delivering care to infants (AAP/Canadian Paediatric Society [CPS], 2000, 2006; IASP, 2005; Joint Commission on Accreditation of Healthcare Organizations [JCAHO], 2001; NANN, 2001).

2. Pain is assessed and reassessed at regular intervals throughout the infant's hospitalization (Agency for Health Care Policy and Research [AHCPR], 1992; AAP/CPS, 2000, 2006; IASP, 2005; JCAHO, 2001; NANN, 2001).

3. Use both nonpharmacologic and pharmacologic therapies to control or prevent pain (AHCPR, 1992; AAP/CPS, 2000, 2006; Anand & International Evidence-Based Group for Neonatal Pain [IEBGNP], 2001; IASP, 2005; NANN, 2001).

4. A collaborative, interdisciplinary approach to pain control should be used by all members of the health care team and infant's family to develop a pain management plan. Include the input of all members of the health care team as well as that of the infant's family whenever possible (AHCPR, 1992; AAP, 1999; IASP, 2005; JCAHO, 2001; NANN, 2001).

5. Pain assessment and management practices should be documented in a manner that facilitates regular reassessment and follow-up intervention (IASP, 2005; JCAHO, 2001).

6. Policies and procedures that support and promote optimal pain assessment and management practices should be established by institutions caring for infants (AHCPR, 1992; AAP/CPS, 2000; JCAHO, 2001).

7. Institutions caring for infants should collect data to monitor the appropriateness and effectiveness of their pain management practices (AHCPR, 1992; IASP, 2005; JCAHO, 2001).

The AAP/APS recommends a comprehensive approach to pediatric pain management, such as increased knowledge of pediatric pain and how to manage it; nonpharmacological measures, such as reducing stimuli and involving the family; using appropriate pain assessment tools and techniques; effective use of pain medication; and increased research and evaluation of analgesics for children (AAP/APS, 2001).

REFERENCES

Adriaensen, H., Gybels, J., Handwerker, H. O., & Van Hees, J. (1983). Response properties of thin myelinated A-delta fibers in human skin nerves. *Journal of Neurophysiology, 49*, 111–122.

Allegaert, K., van den Anker, J. N., & Naulaers, G. (2007). Determinants of drug metabolism in early neonatal life. *Current Clinical Pharmacology, 2*(1), 23–29.

American Academy of Pediatrics. (1987). Neonatal anesthesia. *Pediatrics, 80*(3), 446.

American Academy of Pediatrics and Canadian Paediatric Society. (2006). Prevention and management of pain in the neonate. *Pediatrics, 118*, 2231.

American Academy of Pediatrics Committee on Drugs. (2002). Uses of drugs not described in the package insert (off-label uses). *Pediatrics, 110*, 181–183.

American Academy of Pediatrics, Committee on Fetus and Newborn, Committee on Drugs, Section on Anesthesiology, Section on Surgery, Canadian Paediatric Society, and Fetus and Newborn Committee. (2000). Prevention and management of pain and stress in the neonate. *Pediatrics, 105*(2), 454–461.

American Academy of Pediatrics, Committee on Psychosocial Aspects of Child and Family Health, & Task Force on Pain in Infants, Children, and Adolescents. (2001). The assessment and management of acute pain in infants, children, and adolescents. *Pediatrics, 108*(3), 793–797.

Anand, K. J. S. (1990). Neonatal stress responses to anesthesia and surgery. *Clinics in Perinatology, 17*, 207.

Anand, K. J. S. (1993). Relationship between stress responses and clinical outcomes in newborns, infants and children. *Critical Care Medicine, 21*(9), S358.

Anand, K. J. S. (2007). Pharmacological approaches to the management of pain in the neonatal intensive care unit. *Journal of Perinatology, 27,* S4–S11.

Anand, K. J. S., Aranda, J. V., Berde, C. B., Buckman, S., Capparelli, E. V., Carlo, W., ... Walco, G. A. (2006). Summary proceedings from the neonatal pain-control group. *Pediatrics, 117*(3), S9–S22.

Anand, K. J. S., & Hickey, P. R. (1987). Pain and its effects in the human neonate and fetus. *New England Journal of Medicine, 317,* 1321–1329.

Bartocci, M., Bergqvist, L. L., Lagercrantz, H., & Anand, K. J. S. (2006). Pain activates cortical areas in the preterm newborn brain. *Pain, 122,* 109–117.

Burddeau, G., & Kleiber, C. (1991). Clinical indicators of infant irritability. *Neonatal Network, 9,* 23.

Choonara, I., & Conroy, S. (2002). Unlicensed and off-label drug use in children: Implications for safety. *Drug Safety, 25,* 1–5.

Coderre, T. J., Katz, J., Vaccarino, A. L., & Melzack, R. (1993). Contribution of central neuroplasticity to pathological pain: Review of clinical and experimental evidence. *Pain, 52,* 259–285.

Cope, D. K. (1998, September). Neonatal pain: The evolution of an idea. *American Association of Anesthesiologists Newsletter.* Retrieved from http://anestit.unipa.it/mirror/asa2/newsletters/1998/09_98/Neonatal_0998.html

Darwin, C. (1872). *The expression of the emotions in man and animals* (1st ed.). London, UK: John Murray.

Devor, M. (1994). The pathophysiology of damaged nerves. In P. D. Wall & R. Melzak (Eds.), *Textbook of pain* (3rd ed., pp. 79–100). New York, NY: Churchill Livingstone.

Devor, M. (1996). Pain mechanisms and pain syndromes. In J. Campbell (Ed.), *Pain 1996: An updated review.* Seattle, WA: IASP Press.

Evans, J. C., Vogelpohl, D. G., Bourguignon, C. M., & Morcott, C. S. (1997). Pain behaviors in LBW infants accompany some "non-painful" caregiving procedures. *Neonatal Network, 16,* 33.

Food and Drug Administration. (2001). *The pediatric exclusivity provision: January 2001 status report to Congress.* Rockville, MD: Author.

Gardner, S. L., Carter, B. S., Enzman-Hines, M., & Hernandez, J. A. (2011). *Merenstein & Gardner's handbook of neonatal intensive care* (7th ed.). St. Louis, MO: Mosby.

Hall, R., & Anand, K. J. S. (2005). Physiology of pain and stress in the newborn. *NeoReviews, 6,* 61.

Johnson, C. C., Collinge, J., & Henderson, S. (1997). A cross-sectional survey of pain and pharmacological analgesia in Canadian NICUs. *Clinical Journal of Pain, 13,* 308.

Le, J. (2014). *Drug absorption.* Retrieved from www.merckmanuals.com

McMahon, S. B., Koltzenburg, M., Tracey, I., & Turk, D. C. (2013). *Wall and Melzack's textbook of pain.* Philadelphia, PA: Elsevier Saunders.

Melzack, R., & Wall, P. D. (1965). Pain mechanisms: A new theory. *Science, 150*(3699), 971–979.

Merskey, H. (1979). *Pain, 6,* 250. Retrieved from the International Association for the Study of Pain, http://www.iasp-pain.org/Education/Content.aspx?ItemNumber=1698&&navItemNumber=576#Pain

Merskey, H., Lindblom, U., Mumford, J. M., Nathan, P. W., & Sunderland, S. (1994). Part III: Pain terms, a current list with definitions and notes on usage. In H. Merskey & N. Bogduk (Eds.), *Classification of chronic pain* (2nd ed., pp. 209–214). Seattle, WA: IASP Press.

Meyer, R., Campbell, J., & Raja, S. (1994). Peripheral neural mechanisms of nociception. In P. Wall & R. Melzack (Eds.), *Textbook of pain.* Edinburgh, UK: Churchill Livingstone.

Schecter, N., Berde, C., & Yaster, M. (2002). *Pain in infants, children and adolescents* (2nd ed.). Philadelphia, PA: Lippincott Williams & Wilkins.

Sherrington C. S. (1906). *The integrative action of the nervous system.* New Haven, CT: Yale University Press.

Simons, S., vanDijk, M., Anand, K. S., Roofthooft, D., van Lingen, R. A., & Tibboel, D. (2003). Do we still hurt newborn babies? A prospective study of procedural pain and analgesia in neonates. *Archives of Pediatrics and Adolescent Medicine, 157,* 1058.

Slater, R., Cantarella, A., Gallella, S., Worley, A., Boyd, S., Meek, J., & Fitzgerald, M. (2006). Cortical pain responses in human infants. *Journal of Neuroscience, 26,* 3662–3666.

Stevens, B. (1999). Pain in infants. In M. McCaffery & C. Pasero (Eds.), *Pain: Clinical manual* (2nd ed.). St. Louis, MO: Mosby.

Methods of Assessing Pain in the Newborn

Assessing neonatal pain appropriately is a vital step in providing adequate management of pain. Accurate assessment of pain is challenging in the neonatal population for several reasons. The most obvious is the neonate's inability to verbalize the exact location and intensity of pain along with other verbal descriptors adult patients are able to provide to direct pain management. Gestational age and maturity also inhibit the neonate's ability to provide physiological and physical cues of pain. Because of the subjective nature of pain, the level of skill of the health care worker contributes or detracts from recognizing and assessing pain cues. Subjective observations can change relative to the pain assessment tool used for a particular neonatal environment. A review of physiological cues of neonatal pain beginning with a term newborn through gestational ages in 2-week increments provides a deeper understanding of the presentation of pain symptoms of neonates.

Term, healthy newborns possess a mature neurological system with myelinated neuronal pathways of the neospinothalamic and paleospinothalamic tracts and relatively well-functioning pathways and perceptions (Lowery, Hardman, Manning, Whit Hall, & Anand, 2007). Myelination is sufficiently mature in the sensory, cerebellar, and extrapyramidal tracts, for involuntary reflex and movement for perception and response to painful stimuli. The term newborn's neurological system has an adequate capacity to perceive and respond to tactile stimulation, including pain. Areas most sensitive and thus most mature in term newborns are the face, hands, and soles of the feet. With the capacity to perceive and respond to pain, the term newborn does so through physiological and behavioral cues.

Physiological cues of a healthy term newborn include hormonal, metabolic, and cardiorespiratory changes (Bouwmeester, van Dijk, & Tibboel, n.d.). Hormonal changes affecting cortisol levels vary by gestational age, but tend to fluctuate the least in term newborns (Grunau, 2013). Cortisol levels are important for the newborn's ability to regulate glycolysis and glucose homeostasis. Increasing stress from unrecognized and unmanaged pain will result in cortisol abnormalities even in the healthy term newborn (Heckmann, Wudy, Haack, & Pohlandt, 1999).

Metabolic changes that occur in newborns with poorly managed pain include a propensity for catabolic metabolism. Protein breakdown increases, which contributes to reduced healing capacity. Abnormal nutrient absorption occurs, which contributes to metabolic dysfunction and glucose instability, both of which increase morbidity and mortality from unmanaged pain (Matthew & Matthew, 2003).

Cardiorespiratory changes frequently seen in neonates experiencing pain include bradycardic episodes, decreased oxygenation, ventilation-perfusion mismatch, and increased oxygen consumption. Each of these changes contributes to detrimental outcomes for the infant, ranging from neurological deficits to organ dysfunction.

Bradycardic episodes decrease total circulating volume, reducing perfusion and oxygen delivery to vital organs and tissue. Gastrointestinal perfusion is most significantly affected, compromising digestion and peristalsis. Severe and prolonged bradycardic episodes can lead to reduced renal perfusion, compromising acid–base balance, and clearance of toxins and waste.

Decreased oxygenation and ventilation–perfusion mismatch leads to decreased availability of oxygen at a cellular level, compromising oxygen delivery to tissues and vital organs. Again, gastrointestinal function is most affected, contributing to microscopic areas of infarct, which can contribute to collectively larger areas of infarct and necrotizing enterocolitis. Decreased availability of oxygen is known to lead to cerebral damage and potentially lifelong neurological deficits (Ball & Bindler, 2007; Kenner & Lott, 2003).

The perception of and response to pain increases metabolic energy demands, increasing the cellular need for oxygen availability. When oxygen availability is reduced as a result of bradycardic episodes, the capacity to maintain a higher metabolic energy load is decreased. Increasing oxygen needs with decreasing oxygen availability creates a negative scenario for metabolic and physiologic stability. The infant will resort to anaerobic metabolism at a much quicker rate, increasing lactic acid levels and increasing risks related to anaerobic metabolism (Ball & Bindler, 2007).

As the gestational age of the infant decreases, so does the physiological maturity of the newborn, which, in turn, affects the infant's ability to process and respond to painful stimuli. With each 2-week decrease in gestational age, the capacity of the neonate to maintain physiological stability decreases. The 36- to 38-week-gestation infant has a decreased capacity to maintain cardiorespiratory function with relation to pain, reducing the ability to maintain oxygenation and perfusion. Cortisol levels become increasingly higher, resulting in decreasing glucose stabilization. Catabolic metabolism increases, resulting in greater protein synthesis (Kenner & Lott, 2003).

Subjective observations of neonatal pain focus on the behavioral cues infants present when experiencing pain. Behavioral cues include a spectrum of behaviors, again influenced by gestational age and neurological maturation and capacity to express behavioral changes. The key behavioral cues infants demonstrate when experiencing pain include irritability, posturing, grimacing, eye squeezing, curled tongue, and stretched open mouths (Schellack, 2011; Tietjen, 2001). As gestational age decreases, the ability of the neonate to manifest these behaviors decreases.

Assessment tools are available that recognize and quantify the physiological and behavioral observations as pain values. Each tool uses a variety of assessment parameters and foci to determine a particular pain range so the practitioner can decide on the intervention that best meets the neonate's needs. Each tool provides a comprehensive, complete range for assessing pain; one must use caution in understanding the patient population one is working with to ensure the most appropriate tool is selected.

CRIES

The CRIES (or crying requires increasing oxygen administration, increased vital signs, expression, sleeplessness) tool, shown in Table 2.1, was developed by a neonatal clinical nurse specialist in Columbia, Missouri, for assessing and measuring neonatal postoperative pain. The tool is appropriate for use with infants 6 months or younger in postoperative intensive care units and pediatric care units. Point values are assigned to assessment criteria for each of the areas identified through the CRIES acronym.

Using CRIES begins with an assessment of crying. Understanding that crying is a normal activity of infants, the presence of a high-pitched cry is typically characteristic of pain. The tool requires the practitioner to evaluate the cry and assign a point value based on the characteristics of the cry. Crying is assessed as either not crying, crying but not high pitched, high-pitched crying but consolable, and inconsolable crying. Zero points are awarded for no crying and crying that is not high pitched. One point is awarded for the high-pitched, consolable cry, and two points for inconsolable crying (Krechel & Bindler, 1995).

Alterations in oxygenation determined by pulse oximetry measurement can be related to many things, such as hypoxemia, oversedation, or pulmonary dysfunction. First ruling out alternate causes for changes in oxygenation leads the practitioner to evaluate changes relative to pain. Oxygen consumption increases when pain is experienced, causing the infant to present with decreased oxygen levels. Oxygen requirements are evaluated in three increments with relative point values. Zero points are assigned when no change in oxygenation is noted and no supplemental oxygen is required. One point is awarded when less than or equal to 30% supplemental oxygen is required to maintain oxygen saturation greater than 95%. Two points are

|awarded when less than or equal to 30% supplemental oxygen is required to maintain oxygen saturation greater than 95% (Krechel & Bindler, 1995).

When assessing the vital signs of a previously stable neonate, increasing vital signs' values from pre-operative baseline values indicates an increase in pain. Zero points are assigned when the heart rate and mean blood pressure are less than or equal to the preoperative baseline vital signs. One point is awarded when the heart rate or mean blood pressure increases by less than or equal to 20% from preoperative baseline values. Two points are awarded when the heart rate or mean blood pressure increases greater than 20% from preoperative baseline values. To calculate the evaluation percentage, the baseline heart rate is multiplied by 0.2, and then added to the total baseline value.

Expression assesses behavioral changes with which the infant may present. No expressions, or relaxed, calm facial expressions are awarded zero points. Grimacing receives one point and grimacing with grunting is awarded two points. Grimacing is indicated by a lowered brow, eyes squeezed shut, a deepening of the nasolabial furrow, and open lips and mouth.

Determination of sleeplessness is the last assessment criterion for the CRIES tool. Infants not experiencing any sleeplessness receive zero points. Infants waking at frequent intervals and not enjoying continuous sleep receive one point. Infants who are constantly awake and not enjoying any sleep periods receive two points.

Point values are added from all assessment parameters to create a total score ranging from 0 to 10. The higher the score the infant receives, the greater the subjective assessment of pain expression. Working collaboratively, the health care team determines interventions with the families, if appropriate, in response to the scores (Krechel & Bindler, 1995). A standardized approach to interventions based on scores is imperative prior to using the CRIES tool to ensure consistency and compliance (Krechel, 1995).

TABLE 2.1 CRIES Pain Scale

	DATE/TIME					
Crying—Characteristic cry of pain is high pitched 0—No cry or cry that is not high-pitched 1—Cry high pitched but baby is easily consolable 2—Cry high pitched but baby is inconsolable						
Requires O₂ for SaO₂ < 95%—Babies experiencing pain manifest decreased oxygenation. Consider other causes of hypoxemia, (e.g., oversedation, atelectasis, pneumothorax) 0—No oxygen required 1— < 30% oxygen required 2— > 30% oxygen required						
Increased vital signs (BP and HR)—Take BP last as this may awaken child making other assessments difficult 0—Both HR and BP unchanged or less than baseline 1—HR or BP increased but increases < 20% of baseline 2—HR or BP is increased > 20% over baseline						

Expression—The facial expression most often associated with pain is a grimace. A grimace may be characterized by brow lowering, eyes squeezed shut, deepening naso-labial furrow, or open lips and mouth

0—No grimace present
1—Grimace alone is present
2—Grimace and non-cry vocalization grunt is present

Sleepless—Scored based upon the infant's state during the hour preceding the recorded score

0—Child has been continuously asleep
1—Child has awoken at frequent intervals
2—Child has been awake constantly

TOTAL SCORE

BP, blood pressure; HR, heart rate; SaO$_2$, oxygen saturation.
From Krechel and Bildner (1995). Reprinted with permission.

NEONATAL INFANT PAIN SCALE

The Neonatal Infant Pain Scale (NIPS), as shown in Table 2.2, is a behavioral assessment tool for measuring pain in full-term and preterm infants. Eight indicators assess behaviors believed to be indicative of infant pain and include facial expressions, cry, breathing patterns, arms, legs, and state of arousal. Each indicator has several assessment criteria with point values awarded for each finding. Beginning with facial expression, an infant is assessed as relaxed with a restful, neutral expression, which generates zero points, or grimacing. Grimacing facial expressions are considered to be tight facial muscles, a furrowed brow, chin, and/or jaw, and receive one point.

Crying is assessed as three separate states. No crying, meaning the infant is quiet and calm, receives zero points. Whimpering, mild moaning, and intermittent sounds of discomfort receive one point. Vigorous crying with loud, shrill, continuous screaming receives two points. An infant who is

TABLE 2.2 Neonatal Infant Pain Scale (NIPS)			
NIPS	**0 point**	**1 point**	**2 points**
Facial expression	Relaxed	Contracted	-
Cry	Absent	Mumbling	Vigorous
Breathing	Relaxed	Different than basal	-
Arms	Relaxed	Flexed/stretched	-
Legs	Relaxed	Flexed/stretched	-
Alertness	Sleeping/ calm	Uncomfortable	-

Note: Maximal score of seven points, considering pain ≥ 4.

From Lawrence et al. (1993). Copyright 1993 by Springer Publishing Company. Reprinted with permission.

intubated and crying "silently" can be awarded cry points based on visual assessment of facial expressions and behaviors regardless of sound.

Breathing patterns are assessed as relaxed and usual for the infant being assessed, or as changes in respiration. The infant without any change in normal respiratory movements and patterns receives zero points. The infant with irregular breathing, such as tachypnea, bradypnea, gagging, or apnea, receives one point.

Assessment of arms and legs provides two areas of evaluation and point assignment. Relaxed, smooth movements of arms and legs with no muscle rigidity or posturing noted in either extremity receive zero points for each limb. Infants who hold arms or legs with rigid extension or flexion receive one point for extension of any one of the extremities.

An assessment of the state of arousal again awards the infant zero or one point, based on the assessment findings. An infant who is quietly sleeping or is awake and alert but settled and quietly observing the environment receives zero points. An infant who is fussing, restless, fidgeting, and unable to quietly observe the environment while awake receives one point.

For point value consideration, assessment of heart rate and oxygen saturation require baseline vital signs for comparison. The infant whose heart rate remains within 10% of the documented baseline at all times receives zero points. The infant who requires no supplemental oxygen to maintain oxygen saturation receives zero points. The infant whose heart rate falls within 11% to 20% of the baseline vital signs receives one point. The infant who requires any additional supplemental oxygenation to maintain oxygen saturations at baseline receives one point. The infant whose heart rate exceeds 20% of the documented baselines receives two points, as shown in Table 2.2.

When assessment of the eight criteria is completed, the points awarded are tallied for a total score, indicating a pain level for that individual infant. Any infant scoring greater than three points is considered to be experiencing pain. Practitioners and clinicians need to agree on a comprehensive protocol for interventions to manage pain in increments based on the scores assessed for each infant. A point to consider when using the NIPS assessment tool is not every neonate will have the capacity to present with the assessment criteria in the tool. Infants who are experiencing severe or overwhelming sepsis and/or are receiving paralytic agents as a treatment are unable to manifest the symptoms the clinician is seeking to find. Consideration of contributing factors that will alter the final score are necessary for final pain score determination (Alcock, 1993; Gallo, 2003).

NEONATAL PAIN, AGITATION, AND SEDATION SCALE

The Neonatal Pain, Agitation, and Sedation Scale (N-PASS) is a tool used to measure pain in term and preterm infants who are experiencing prolonged postoperative pain and/or pain during mechanical ventilation. The tool uses five physiological and behavioral cues with relative validity for measurement (Hummel, Puchalski, Creech, & Weiss, 2008). The tool uses an ordinal system for point assessment, with values ranging from minus two to two. N-PASS also considers sedation as an assessment parameter, as shown in Table 2.3. Beginning with crying and irritability, the practitioner first considers the state of sedation of the infant based on pharmaceutical delivery and considers whether the infant has no cry with painful stimuli, and, if so, awards minus two points. The infant who is sedated and elicits minimal moaning or crying with painful stimuli is awarded minus one point. An infant displaying appropriate crying for the situation and is not irritable receives zero points. The infant who is irritable or crying intermittently yet is consolable will receive one point. The infant experiencing high-pitched crying that is continuous or who is intubated and experiences silent continuous crying and is inconsolable will receive two points.

Table 2.3 shows assessment of the behavior state again begins with consideration of the sedation state with minus two points awarded to the infant who exhibits no arousal to any stimuli and exhibits no spontaneous movements. The infant who is sedated and can exhibit minimal arousal to stimuli and has little spontaneous movement will receive minus one point. An infant whose behavior state is appropriate for gestational age receives zero points. The infant who is restless, squirming, and awakens frequently between sleep cycles will earn one point. The infant who is arching, kicking, constantly awake with no sleep cycles or arouses minimally with no movement without sedation is awarded two points (Hummel et al., 2008).

Evaluation of facial expressions begins again with consideration of sedated state, with minus two points awarded when the infant expresses a lax mouth with no expression and minus one point when exhibiting minimal expressions with stimulation. The normal, nonsedated infant experiencing no pain who is relaxed and appropriate for gestational age receives zero points. When evaluating the infant, discovery of any pain expression, even intermittently, earns the infant one point. The infant expressing continual pain through facial expressions receives two points.

Extremities are assessed for reflex expression and tone, as well as posturing behaviors using N-PASS. An infant who is sedated and demonstrating no grasp reflex and whose muscle tone is flaccid will earn minus two points. If the infant is sedated and can demonstrate a weak grasp with decreased muscle tone, minus one point is awarded. The infant without sedation who has relaxed hands and feet with normal tone will earn zero points. The infant who exhibits intermittent clenched toes, fists, or demonstrates finger splaying but whose body is not tense will earn one point. The infant who is continually clenching fists or toes and splaying fingers while also holding his or her body tense will earn two points, as shown in Table 2.3.

TABLE 2.3 N-PASS Pain Scale

N-PASS: Neonatal Pain, Agitation, & Sedation Scale

Assessment Criteria	Sedation		Sedation/Pain	Pain/Agitation	
	-2	-1	0/0	1	2
Crying Irritability	No cry with painful stimuli	Moans or cries minimally with painful stimuli	No sedation/ No pain signs	Irritable or crying at intervals Consolable	High-pitched or silent-continuous cry Inconsolable
Behavior State	No arousal to any stimuli No spontaneous movement	Arouses minimally to stimuli Little spontaneous movement	No sedation/ No pain signs	Restless, squirming Awakens frequently	Arching, kicking Constantly awake or Arouses minimally/no movement (not sedated)

Facial Expression	Mouth is lax No expression	Minimal expression with stimuli	No sedation/ No pain signs	Any pain expression intermittent	Any pain expression continual
Extremities Tone	No grasp reflex Flaccid tone	Weak grasp reflex ↓ muscle tone	No sedation/ No pain signs	Intermittent clenched toes, fists or finger splay Body is not tense	Continual clenched toes, fists, or finger splay Body is tense
Vital signs HR, RR, BP, SaO$_2$	No variability with stimuli Hypoventilation or apnea	< 10% variability from baseline with stimuli	No sedation/ No pain signs	↑ 10%–20% from baseline SaO$_2$ 76%–85% with stimulation—quick ↑	↑ > 20% from baseline SaO$_2$ ≤ 75% with stimulation—slow ↑ Out of sync/fighting vent

Premature Pain Assessment ➤ + 1 if < 30 weeks gestation/corrected age

BP, blood pressure; HR, heart rate, RR, respiratory rate; SaO$_2$, oxygen saturation.

ASSESSMENT OF SEDATION

■ Sedation is scored in addition to pain for each behavioral and physiological criteria to assess the infant's response to stimuli

■ Sedation does not need to be assessed/scored with every pain assessment/score

■ Sedation is scored from $0 \rightarrow -2$ for each behavioral and physiological criteria, then summed and noted as a negative score ($0 \rightarrow -10$)

■ A score of 0 is given if the infant has no signs of sedation, does not under-react

■ Desired levels of sedation vary according to the situation

■ "Deep sedation" $\rightarrow$ goal score of -10 to -5

■ "Light sedation" $\rightarrow$ goal score of -5 to -2

■ Deep sedation is not recommended unless an infant is receiving ventilatory support, related to the high potential for hypoventilation and apnea

ASSESSMENT OF PAIN/AGITATION

■ Pain assessment is the fifth vital sign – assessment for pain should be included in every vital sign assessment

■ Pain is scored from $0 \rightarrow +2$ for each behavioral and physiological criteria, then summed

■ Points are added to the premature infant's pain score based on the gestational age to compensate for the limited ability to behaviorally communicate pain

■ Total pain score is documented as a positive number ($0 \rightarrow +11$)

■ Treatment/interventions are suggested for scores > 3

■ Interventions for known pain/painful stimuli are indicated before the score reaches 3

■ The goal of pain treatment/intervention is a score ≤ 3

■ More frequent pain assessment indications

■ Indwelling tubes or lines which may cause pain, especially with movement (e.g. chest tubes) $\rightarrow$ at least every 2–4 hours

- A negative score without the administration of opioids/sedatives may indicate:
  - The premature infant's response to prolonged or persistent pain/stress
  - Neurologic depression, sepsis, or other pathology

- Receiving analgesics and/or sedatives → at least every 2–4 hours
- 30-60 minutes after an analgesic is given for pain behaviors to assess response to medication
- Post-operative → at least every 2 hours for 24–48 hours, then every 4 hours until off medications

Paralysis/Neuromuscular Blockade

- It is impossible to behaviorally evaluate a paralyzed infant for pain
- Increases in heart rate and blood pressure at rest or with stimulation may be the only indicator of a need for more analgesia
- Analgesics should be administered continuously by drip or around-the-clock dosing
  - Higher, more frequent doses may be required if the infant is post-op, has a chest tube, or other pathology (such as NEC) that would normally cause pain
  - Opioid doses should be increased by 10% every 3-5 days as tolerance will occur without symptoms of inadequate analgesia

SCORING CRITERIA

CRYING/IRRITABILITY

−2 → No response to painful stimuli

- No cry with needle sticks
- No reaction to ETT or nares suctioning
- No response to care giving

−1 → Moans, sighs, or cries (audible or silent) minimally to painful stimuli, e.g. needle sticks, ETT or nares suctioning, care giving

0 → No sedation signs or no pain/agitation signs

+1 → Infant is irritable/crying at intervals—but can be consoled

- If intubated—intermittent silent cry

+2 → Any of the following

- Cry is high-pitched
- Infant cries inconsolably
- If intubated—silent continuous cry

EXTREMITIES/TONE

−2 → Any of the following

- No palmar or plantar grasp can be elicited
- Flaccid tone

−1 → Any of the following

- Weak palmar or plantar grasp can be elicited
- Decreased tone

0 → No sedation signs or No pain/agitation signs

+1 → Intermittent (< 30 seconds duration) observation of toes and/or hands as clenched, or fingers splayed

- Body is *not* tense

+2 → Any of the following

- Frequent (≥ 30 seconds duration) observation of toes and/or hands as clenched, or fingers splayed
- Body is tense/stiff

BEHAVIOR/STATE

−2 →Does not arouse or react to any stimuli

- Eyes continually shut or open
- No spontaneous movement

−1 →Little spontaneous movement, arouses briefly and/or minimally to any stimuli

- Opens eyes briefly
- Reacts to suctioning
- Withdraws to pain

0 →No sedation signs or No pain/agitation signs

+1 →Any of the following

- Restless, squirming
- Awakens frequently/easily with minimal or no stimuli

+2 →Any of the following

- Kicking
- Arching

VITAL SIGNS: HR, BP, RR, & O$_2$ SATURATIONS

−2 →Any of the following

- No variability in vital signs with stimuli
- Hypoventilation
- Apnea
- Ventilated infant—no spontaneous respiratory effort

−1 →Vital signs show little variability with stimuli—less than 10% from baseline

0 →No sedation signs or No pain/agitation signs

+1 →Any of the following

- HR, RR, and/or BP are 10–20% above baseline
- With care/stimuli infant desaturates minimally to moderately (SaO$_2$ 76–85%) and recovers quickly (within 2 minutes)

+2 →Any of the following

- HR, RR, and/or BP are > 20% above baseline

- Constantly awake
- No movement or minimal arousal with stimulation (not sedated, inappropriate for gestational age or clinical situation)

- With care/stimuli infant desaturates severely ($SaO_2 < 75\%$) and recovers slowly (> 2 minutes)
- Out of sync/fighting ventilator

© Loyola University Health System, Loyola University Chicago (2009). Pat Hummel, MA, APN, NNP, PNP. Reprinted with permission.

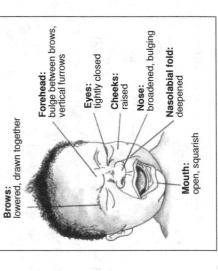

Facial expression of physical distress and pain in the infant.
Reproduced with permission from Wong DL, Hess CS: Wong and Whaley's Clinical Manual of Pediatric Nursing, Ed. 5, 2000, Mosby, St. Louis

FACIAL EXPRESSION

−2 → Any of the following

- Mouth is lax
- Drooling
- No facial expression at rest or with stimuli

−1 → Minimal facial expression with stimuli

0 → No sedation signs or No pain/agitation signs

+1 → Any pain face expression observed intermittently

+2 → Any pain face expression is continual

When evaluating vital signs with N-PASS, assessment of heart rate, respiration, blood pressure, and pulse oximetry are necessary. The sedated infant who shows no variability from baseline with any stimuli or is hypoventilated or experiencing apneic episodes will earn minus two points. The sedated infant who experiences up to but less than 10% variability from baseline vital signs with any stimuli earns minus one point. The infant who enjoys vital signs that remain within baseline for gestational age receives zero points. The infant who has an increase in baseline vital signs from 10% to 20% and exhibits pulse oximetry readings between 76% and 85% with quick recovery with stimulation earns one point. The infant who exhibits an increase in vital signs greater than 20% from baseline with pulse oximetry readings equal to or less than 75% and is slow to recover or is out of synchronization with ventilator support earns two points (Hummel et al., 2003).

When all assessment criteria in all areas are complete, a number value is calculated. To ensure premature infants' pain is adequately captured using N-PASS, providers compensate for decreased capacity of the infant to exhibit physiological and behavioral cues by adding points to the total score. For infants less than 28 weeks gestation, the practitioner must add three points; for the infant less than 28 to 31 weeks gestation, add two points; and the infant less than 32 to 35 weeks gestation, add one point to the total score. The total score is documented as a whole number ranging from 0 to 10. The infant is considered to be experiencing pain that requires intervention when scores exceed a value of three. The goal is to maintain total pain scores below three for any infant. Interventions and management of scores greater than three will require a collaborative and comprehensive intervention plan that is adhered to for all infants (Hummel et al., 2003).

PREMATURE INFANT PAIN PROFILE

The Premature Infant Pain Profile (PIPP) is a pain assessment tool that measures behavioral expression of pain in neonates, especially for premature infants, as highlighted in Table 2.4. The

TABLE 2.4 Premature Infant Pain Profile

Indicators	0	1	2	3
GA in weeks	≥ 36 weeks	32 to 35 weeks and 6 days	28 to 31 weeks and 6 days	< 28 weeks
Observe the NB for 15sec				
Alertness	Active Awake Opened eyes Facial movements present	Quiet Awake Opened eyes No facial movements	Active Sleep Closed eyes Facial movements present	Quiet Sleeping Closed eyes No facial movements
Record HR and SpO$_2$				
Maximal HR	↑ 0 to 4 bpm	↑ 5 to 14 bpm	↑ 15 to 24 bpm	↑ ≥ 25 bpm
Minimal Saturation	↓ 0 to 2.4%	↓ 2.5 to 4.9%	↓ 5 to 7.4%	↓ ≥7.5%
Observe NB for 30 sec				
Frowned forehead	Absent	Minimal	Moderate	Maximal

| Eyes squeezed | Absent | Minimal | Moderate | Maximal |
| Nasolabial furrow | Absent | Minimal | Moderate | Maximal |

Absent is defined as 0 to 9% of the observation time; minimal, 10% to 39% of the time; moderate, 40% to 69% of the time; and maximal as 70% or more of the observation time. In this scale, scores vary from zero to 21 points. Scores equal or lower than 6 indicate absence of pain or minimal pain; scores above 12 indicate the presence of moderate to severe pain.

BPM, beats per minute; GA, gestational age; HR, heart rate; NB, newborn.

From Stevens, Johnston, Petryshen, and Taddio (1996). Reprinted with permission.

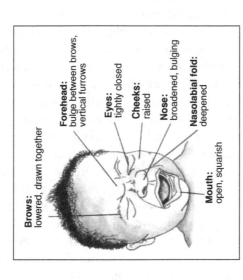

Facial expression of physical distress and pain in the infant.

Reproduced with permission from Wong DL, Hess CS: Wong and Whaley's Clinical Manual of Pediatric Nursing, Ed. 5, 2000, Mosby, St. Louis

tool evaluates seven criteria, awarding points to assessment findings. The tool evaluates gestational age, behavioral state before painful stimulus, and the changes in physiological states during painful stimulus, and physical behaviors of the infant during painful stimulus. The infant must be assessed and receive a baseline score as well as baseline vital signs prior to the painful event to accurately assess response to pain. Gestational age is assessed and awarded point as zero for equal to or greater than 36 weeks, one point for a gestational age of 32 to 35 weeks and 6 days, and two points for 28 weeks to 31 weeks and 6 days gestation (Walden & Gibbins, 2008).

For behavioral state, zero points are awarded for an infant who is active and awake, whose eyes are open, and who has appropriate facial movements. The infant who is quiet and awake, with eyes open, and no facial movements earns one point. The infant who is active or sleeping with eyes closed and has facial movements earns two points. The infant who is quiet or sleeping with eyes closed and no facial movements noted within a 15-second assessment time, earns three points (Walden & Gibbins, 2008).

The heart rate assessment compares the 15 seconds prior to and during painful stimulus to the baseline findings previously documented by the clinician. Heart rate increases of zero to four beats above baseline will earn zero points. Heart rate increases of five to 14 beats above baseline earn one point. An increase in heart rate of 15 to 24 beats above baseline earns two points; an increase of equal to or greater than 25 beats from baseline earns three points.

Oxygen saturation assessment also compares the 15-second baseline assessment to and during the painful stimuli assessment findings. Increases in oxygen saturation from 0% to 2.4% earn zero points. An increase ranging from 2.5% to 4.95% earns one point. Increases that range from 5% to 7.4% will earn two points and increases greater than 7.5% will earn three points.

Consideration of brow bulging assesses the squeezing of the eyebrows together and is assessed as a percentage of time the infant holds that facial expression. Eye squeezing refers to the infant purposefully holding the eyes shut. Nasolabial furrow is the creasing or frowning expression of the infant while also attempting to keep eyes squeezed shut. All three assessment criteria are evaluated by visual inspection and need to follow the same time-period considerations for an accurate assessment. The length of time for assessing the behaviors is 30 seconds after the painful stimuli and a calculation of the amount of that time the infant displays the behavior is used to determine a point value. The infant who never displays a brow bulge, eye squeeze, or nasolabial furrow that is equal to or less than 9% of the time receives a zero for each behavior. The infant who displays a brow bulge, eye squeeze, or nasolabial furrow 10% to 39% of the time or minimally, receives one point for each behavior. The infant who displays a brow bulge, eye squeeze, or nasolabial furrow 40% to 69% of the time or moderately, receives two points for each behavior. The infant who displays the brow bulge, eye squeeze, or nasolabial furrowing behavior equal to or greater than 70% receives three points for each behavior, as noted in Table 2.4 (Walden & Gibbins, 2008).

FACE, LEGS, ACTIVITY, CRY, AND CONSOLABILITY SCALE

The Face, Legs, Activity, Cry, and Consolability (FLACC) pain scale, shown in Table 2.5, is a behavioral pain assessment tool useful for measuring postoperative pain in young children. The tool has each of the five categories described by FLACC. Each category has three scoring possibilities from zero to two. The patient should be assessed from 1 to 5 minutes or longer when awake, with legs and body uncovered. If necessary, the patient can be repositioned and observed after he or she has settled, while assessing the entire body for tension and tone. The infant who is sleeping should be observed for 5 minutes or longer when using the FLACC scale. The patient's legs and

TABLE 2.5 FLACC Pain Scale

Categories	Scoring		
	0	1	2
Face	No particular expression or smile; disinterested	Occasional grimace or frown, withdrawn	Frequent to constant frown, clenched jaw, quivering chin
Legs	Normal position or relaxed	Uneasy, restless, tense	Kicking, or legs drawn up
Activity	Lying quietly, normal position, moves easily	Squirming, shifting back and forth, tense	Arched, rigid, or jerking
Cry	No cry (awake or asleep)	Moans or whimpers, occasional complaint	Crying steadily, screams or sobs, frequent complaints
Consolability	Content, relaxed	Reassured by occasional touching, hugging, or talked to. Distractable	Difficult to console or comfort

Each of the five categories (F) Face; (L) Legs; (A) Activity; (C) Cry; (C) Consolability is scored from 0–2, which results in a total score between 0 and 10.

The FLACC scale was developed by Sandra Merkel, MS, RN; Terri Voepel-Lewis, MS, RN; and Shobha Malviya, MD, at C. S. Mott Children's Hospital, University of Michigan Health System, Ann Arbor, MI. Used with permission. Copyright the Regents of the University of Michigan.

body should be uncovered, and, if necessary, touch the patient to observe for tension and tone in response. When determining a score assignment, each category should be observed and a determination of actions made.

When assessing the face, a zero is awarded if the patient has no expression, makes eye contact if awake, and shows an interest in the surroundings. A score of one is assigned if the patient demonstrates an occasional grimace or frown awake or asleep, is withdrawn or disinterested with a worried facial expression when awake, has eyebrows lowered and eyes partially closed, cheeks raised, and mouth pursed awake or asleep. To earn a score of two, the patient must demonstrate deep furrows in the forehead, have a clenched jaw, quivering lips, open mouth, deep lines around the nose and lips in sleep and when awake (Jacques, 2015).

Assessing the legs begins with assessment of movement. If legs are in a normal resting position and relaxed, with normal tone, a zero is assigned. A score of one is earned if the legs are uneasy, restless, or tense in sleep or awake, have increased tone or rigidity, and if intermittent flexion or extension is noted. A score of two is assigned if the child demonstrates hypertonicity, legs pulled tight with exaggerated flexion or extension, trembling, and kicking or drawing up of the legs.

Activity assessment begins with state assessment. Is the child lying quietly, in a normal position, moving easily and freely without restrictions? A score of zero is awarded. The child who is squirming, shifting back and forth, is tense, appears to hesitate before moving, demonstrates guarding, has a tense torso, or hesitates placing pressure on a body part receives a one. A child who is arched, has rigid tone, is in a fixed position, demonstrates side-to-side head movement, or is rubbing a particular body part receives a two (Jacques, 2015).

When assessing the cry of the child, a zero is awarded to the child who is content, relaxed, not crying or moaning, whether awake or asleep. A two is assigned to the child who is moaning or whimpering, has an occasional complaint verbalized in appropriate terminology for the age, or is sighing frequently.

A three is awarded to the child who is crying steadily, screams or sobs, has frequent complaints, or is grunting.

Finally, to assess consolability, the caregiver determines whether the infant is content and relaxed, is calm, and does not require any consoling. If so, a score of zero is assigned. A child who is reassured with occasional touching, hugging, or soft talking, who is distracted from discomfort within 30 seconds to 1 minute, earns a score of one. A child who is difficult or unable to be consoled or comforted and who requires constant attention earns a two (Jacques, 2015).

Ideally, self-reporting from the child is necessary in combination with observed behaviors. If self-reporting is not possible, careful consideration of the assessment findings in the context of the pain findings is necessary before making decisions about appropriate interventions. Once all categories are assessed and a resulting score of zero to 10 is achieved, determination of the degree of pain is made. A score of zero is relaxed and comfortable, with no apparent pain and no interventions necessary. A score of one to three indicates mild discomfort and repositioning or distraction is necessary. A score of four to six reveals moderate pain and requires some intervention of distraction, consoling, repositioning, or pharmaceuticals. A score of seven to 10 indicates severe discomfort and/or pain and requires pharmaceutical intervention.

LEVELS OF SEDATION

Level of sedation in pediatric patients poses special problems with identifying pain and providing appropriate pain relief. The American Academy of Pediatrics established criteria for determination of levels of sedation for monitoring the child's vital signs and for determining the level of observation and care required for the sedated child. In 2006, the Joint Commission on Accreditation of Healthcare Organizations, the American Society of Anesthesiologists, and the American Academy of Pediatrics updated the terminology and categories of sedation for pediatric patients to ensure all associations are using the same comprehensive standards. Sedation alters the ability to assess pain properly in the pediatric population and standardized definitions are necessary to provide appropriate interventions. The age and developmental stage of the child further complicates the ability to assess pain correctly; therefore, an understanding of the levels of sedation is imperative to assess pain competently. As such, *minimal, moderate*, and *deep sedation* are defined using the following criteria.

Minimal sedation is considered anxiolysis, or a state of reduced anxiety. Infant responsiveness to stimuli is appropriate—meaning pain reflexes, guarding, and developmentally appropriate responses to stimuli still occur during minimal sedation. The ability to maintain effective ventilation without respiratory or cardiovascular support in terms of airway maintenance is still independent. The infant under minimal sedation requires observation and intermittent assessment to ensure continued airway independence and appropriate stimuli response by a registered nurse or physician (Sheta, 2010).

Moderate sedation is what was previously called *conscious sedation*. The infant is still "conscious," that is, the infant still has a purposeful response to light stimuli, has the ability to maintain an airway independently, and has adequate independent ventilation. Cardiovascular support is not necessary with conscious sedation. Vital-sign monitoring is necessary for the infant experiencing moderate sedation. Continuous pulse oximetry, continuous heart rate, and respiratory monitoring are necessary, as are intermittent blood pressure readings. One-to-one observation by a registered nurse or physician should be maintained throughout the conscious sedation; with access to other support, personnel should check the stability of the infant for change at any time during the sedated state (Sheta, 2010).

Deep sedation, as described by the American Academy of Pediatrics, is a deep sleep state in which the infant can still exhibit a purposeful response to painful stimuli. The infant requires support or intervention to maintain an airway, has no independent capacity for ventilation, and requires cardiovascular support during deep sedation. Monitoring of the infant requires continuous pulse oximetry, cardiac monitoring, and continuous blood pressure monitoring. An infant experiencing

TABLE 2.6 Levels of Sedation			
Descriptor	Minimal Sedation	Moderate Sedation	Deep Sedation
Pain reflex	Responsive to tactile, deep stimuli	Responsive to tactile, deep stimuli	Responsive to tactile, deep stimuli
Cardiovascular	Spontaneous, does not require support	Spontaneous, does not require support	Spontaneous, may not require support
Respiratory	Spontaneous respirations	Spontaneous respirations	Some spontaneous respirations; requires support
Oxygenation	Maintained	May require supplemental FiO_2	Requires supplemental oxygenation
Nursing support	Observation	Observation	Supportive

Fio$_2$, fraction of inspired oxygen.
Source: Sheta (2010).

deep sedation requires one-to-one monitoring by a licensed professional, with support personnel immediately available for interventions (Sheta, 2010). Table 2.6 details all levels of sedation and describes each level for easy reference.

EFFECTIVENESS OF PAIN MANAGEMENT

The effectiveness of pain management requires an understanding of the behavioral cues of the infant and a working knowledge of the pain tool being used. Understanding the developmental differences of the gestational age of the infant is necessary for adequately assessing pain and assessing response to interventions to resolve pain. Behavioral clues, such as sleep state, vital-sign stability, and stimuli response, vary with gestational age. Caretaker observation and knowledge of infant's "usual" behaviors are also necessary for adequate pain assessment. Obtaining baseline behavior cues, such as sleep state, vital-sign stability, and consolability, as well as stress behaviors is imperative in understanding the effectiveness of interventions.

Assessment of behavioral cues, such as sleep state and awake states, is a necessary part of assessing effectiveness of pain management. Sleep states include quiet sleep and active sleep. Quiet sleep is a deep state of rest that is restorative and anabolic—meaning a time of growth and maintenance. The tissues and organs are moving to a reparative state or growing and differentiating to a mature state. The infant in quiet sleep is nearly still, with the occasional startle or twitch while remaining asleep. In quiet sleep, there is no recognizable eye movement or facial movements. An infant in quiet sleep will have occasional sucking motions, but remains still and asleep. The breathing patterns of quiet sleep are even and regular, with oxygen saturation maintained without disruption. The infant in quiet sleep is not easily roused, exhibiting responses only to very intense and disturbing stimuli, such as extreme pain. Infants in a quiet sleep state are not easily responsive and tend to return to this state even after disturbing stimuli (Blackburn & Blackwell-Sachs, 2003).

The infant spends the longest portion of his or her sleep time in active sleep. During active sleep, processing and storing of information occurs, and is believed to be the time when sleep is linked to learning. The active sleep state typically precedes wakening. An infant in active sleep or rapid eye movement (REM) sleep has some body movements—primarily limb readjustment for self-comfort. REM is noted during active sleep, with the eyes fluttering beneath closed lids but no actual eye opening. An infant in active sleep may smile and may exhibit soft crying. Breathing patterns during active sleep are irregular, but oxygen saturations are maintained without disruption. An infant in active sleep is responsive to internal stimuli cues, such as hunger, and external cues such as touch or noise. The infant in active sleep will respond to the stimuli and continue to a wakeful state or return to active sleep or even transition back to quiet sleep (Blackburn & Blackwell-Sachs, 2003).

The behaviors of the awake state include drowsy, quiet alert, active alert, and crying. Infants in a drowsy state exhibit variable movements with mild startle intermingled with activity and movements that are usually smooth and controlled. The eyes occasionally open and close, but are heavy lidded or slitted. The infant in a drowsy state may have some facial movement, but generally has none, and the face will appear still most of the time. The breathing pattern is irregular, but no changes in oxygen saturation will be evident. The infant will react to sensory stimuli during a drowsy state, but reactions may be delayed. The infant will transition to quiet alert, active alert, or crying after sensory stimulus. If the sensory stimulus is removed, the infant may return to sleep state without difficulty (Blackburn & Blackwell-Sachs, 2003).

In a quiet alert state, the infant has minimal body activity with limited movements of any extremity. The eyes are bright and widened, taking in the environment. The infant has an attentive appearance during the quiet alert state, seemingly taking in the stimulus and environment. Breathing is regular, with no changes in oxygen saturation. Infants in the quiet alert state are most attentive during this state, readily processing stimuli and focusing on the environment.

In the active alert state, the infant exhibits variable activity, from mild startles to stimulus intermingled with movements that remain smooth and controlled. The eyes are open during the active alert state, but have a dull, glazed appearance. The facial movements during are minimal; most likely there will be no movements and the face will remain still without expression. Breathing is irregular during the active alert state, without any changes in oxygen saturation. During the active alert state, the infant will react to sensory stimulus, but again, reactions may be delayed. The infant is likely to transition to a quiet alert or crying state after sensory input during this state.

During a crying state, the infant has increasing motor activity and skin color is likely to change to a red, ruddy, or darkened color. The eyes may be open or held tightly closed. Grimaces are the facial movements frequently seen during the crying state. Breathing is most irregular during the crying state than in other states and oxygen saturation may be affected. During the crying state, infants are especially sensitive and responsive to unpleasant external or internal stimuli, which signifies that the infant has reached his or her capacity for processing the stimulus (Blackburn & Blackwell-Sachs, 2003).

Assessing vital signs as a method of measuring effectiveness of pain management requires documentation of baseline vital signs prior to negative stimulus. Assessment of the infant during any state other than crying will provide the practitioner a baseline for comparison of changes in vital signs when an unpleasant stimulus is introduced. Many of the pain assessment tools require observation of vital signs for a prescribed amount of time and documentation of those vital signs at the beginning of the care period. Changes that exceed 10% of the baseline vital signs are indicative of a decreasing capacity to process negative stimulus.

Consolability, or the ability to support the infant from a negative state of stimulus to a calmer state, is a measure of how intense or negative the stimulus is for the infant. Different methods of consolability can help the infant achieve the transition, from removing the negative stimulus, to containment, and then to pharmaceutical intervention. Removing negative stimulus can be as simple as removing noxious odors such as alcohol pads, to ending a painful procedure such as a heel stick. Providing containment with boundaries, such as holding or swaddling, can be a simple method of consolation that will allow an infant to transition to a more stable state. When measuring the degree of support, an infant is able to move to a more stable state through consoling and intervention methods, as captured using pain assessment tools (Blackburn & Blackwell-Sachs, 2003).

CONCERNS/LIMITATIONS OF ASSESSING PAIN

The concerns and limitations of assessing pain in the neonatal population are many. Neonates cannot provide a verbal report of pain or respond to interventions to relieve pain and a practitioner must rely on objective factors and physiological cues to arrive at an estimate of pain. Objective factors can inhibit the accurate assessment of initial pain values and infant responses to interventions relative to experience and attentiveness. Physiological cues can be objective when considering the gestational age and neurological maturity of an infant. The less mature the infant, the less able he or she is to exhibit physiological changes indicative of pain. Physiological alterations caused by disease states can alter the infant's presentation and ability to exhibit changes in state as well. Astute and frequent assessments of the infant are necessary to accurately evaluate and monitor pain and the infant's response to interventions to reduce pain so as to enhance the infant's neurological and developmental outcomes.

REFERENCES

Alcock, L. J. (1993). The development of a tool to assess neonatal pain. *Neonatal Network, 12*(6), 59–66.

Ball, J., & Bindler, R. (2007). *Pediatric nursing: Caring for children* (4th ed.). Upper Saddle River, NJ: Pearson Prentice Hall.

Blackburn, S., & Blackwell-Sachs. (2003). *Understanding the behavior of term infants.* White Plains, NY: March of Dimes Birth Defects Foundation.

Bouwmeester, J., van Dijk, M., & Tibboel, D. (n.d.). Human neonates and pain. *Humane endpoints in animal experiments for biomedical research.* Retrieved from http://www.lal.org.uk/uploads/editor/HEP_BOUWMEESTER.pdf

Gallo, A. M. (2003). The fifth vital sign: Implementation of neonatal infant pain scale. *Journal of Obstetric, Gynecologic, and Neonatal Nursing, 32,* 206. doi:10.1177/0884217503251745

Grunau, R. E. (2013). Neonatal pain in very preterm infants: Long-term effects on brain, neurodevelopment and pain reactivity. *Rambam Maimonides Medical Journal, 4*(4), e0025. doi:10.504/RMMJ.10132

Heckmann, M., Wudy, S., Haack, D., & Pohlandt, F. (1999). Reference range for serum cortisol in well preterm infants. *ADC Fetal and Neonatal Edition, 81*(3), F171–F174.

Hummel, P., Puchalski, M., Creech, S. D., & Weiss, M. G. (2008). Clinical reliability and validity of the N-PASS: Neonatal Pain, Agitation, and Sedation Scale with prolonged pain. *Journal of Perinatology, 28,* 55–60. Retrieved from http://www.nature.com/jp/journal/v28/n1/full/7211861a.html

Jacques, E. (2015). *FLACC scale: Pain assessment tool.* Retrieved from http://pain.about.com/od/testingdiagnosis/ig/pain-scales/Flacc-Scale.htm

Kenner, C., & Lott, J. W. (2003). *Comprehensive neonatal nursing: A physiological perspective* (3rd ed.). St. Louis, MO: Saunders.

Krechel, S. W., & Bindler, J. (1995). CRIES: A new neonatal postoperative pain measurement score-initial testing of validity and reliability. *Paediatric Anaesthesia, 5,* 53–61.

Lawrence, J., Alcock, D., McGrath, P., Kay, J., MacMurray, S., & Dulberg, C. (1993). The development of a tool to assess neonatal pain. *Neonatal Network, 12*(6), 59–66.

Lowery, C. L., Hardman, M. P., Manning, N., Whit Hall, R., & Anand, K. J. S. (2007). Neurodevelopmental changes of fetal pain. *Seminars in Perinatology, 31,* 275–282.

Matthew, P. J., & Matthew, J. L. (2003). Assessment and management of pain in infants. *Postgraduate Medical Journal, 79,* 438–443. doi:10.1136/pmj.79.934.438

Schellack, N. (2011). A review of pain management in the neonate. *South African Pharmacy Journal, 78*(7), 10–13.

Sheta, S. A. (2010). Procedural sedation analgesia. *Saudi Journal of Anaesthesia, 4*(1), 11–16. doi:10.4103/16588-351X.62608

Stevens, B., Johnston, C., Petryshen, P., & Taddio, A. (1996). Premature Infant Pain Profile: Development and initial validation. *Clinical Journal of Pain, 12,* (22), 13–22.

Tietjen, S. D. (2001). *Consistent pain assessment in the neonatal intensive care unit.* Retrieved from http://www.vachss.com/guest_dispatches/neonatal_pain.html

Voepel-Lewis, T., Merkel, S., Tait, A. R., Trzcinka, A., & Malviya, S. (2002). The reliability and validity of the FLACC Observational Tool as a measure of pain in children with cognitive impairment. *Anesthesia & Analgesia, 95,* 1224–1229.

Walden, M., & Gibbins, S. (2008). *Pain assessment and management guideline for practice* (2nd ed.). Glenview, IL: National Association of Neonatal Nurses.

Pharmacological Management of Acute and Chronic Pain

3

General Principles of Pain Management

There are several different pharmacological options used to treat neonates who are experiencing pain or undergoing a painful procedure. These treatments generally involve opioids, nonopioids, or coanalgesics.

Opioids are natural, endogenous or synthetic compounds that primarily activate the mu receptors. The term *opiate* refers to a class of alkaloid compounds derived naturally from the poppy, such as morphine and codeine. Heroin, oxycodone, hydromorphone, methadone, and buprenorphine are examples of synthetic opioids (Ries, Fiellin, Miller, & Saitz, 2009). Nonopioids, such as nonsteriodal anti-inflammatory drugs (NSAIDs), among others, refer to drugs that do not bind to opioid receptors. Some may be given with opioids for enhanced effect. Coanalgesics are drugs that do not produce much or any analgesic effect but work to enhance analgesic drugs or offer symptom relief, which leads to pain reduction. These three classifications of medications are discussed specifically in the next chapters and are listed in Table 3.1.

PHARMACOKINETICS AND PHARMACODYNAMICS OF PAIN THERAPY IN NEONATES

Pain can be managed through pharmacological and nonpharmacological means. Although nonpharmacological treatment is preferred in this population, medication is necessary for many of the invasive procedures performed in the neonatal intensive care unit (NICU). The problem with pharmacological measures in the

TABLE 3.1 Modified Drug Classification Reference Table From the Children's Hospital Association

Classification	Examples	Mechanism of Action	Indications	Dosage Considerations	Possible Adverse Effects*
Opioids	Morphine Hydromorphone Codeine Hydrocodone Oxycodone Fentanyl Methadone	Binds to the opioid receptors in the brain and spinal cord during the transmission process	Moderate to severe pain	Titrate to effect (desired analgesia) or intolerable side effects (respiratory depression)	Respiratory depression, nausea, vomiting, constipation, sedation, and urinary retention
Nonopioids	Acetaminophen Aspirin Ibuprofen Naproxen Ketorolac	Inhibits prostaglandin production during the transduction process	Mild to moderate pain, opioidsparing effect, pain secondary to inflammatory conditions	Nonopioids have a "ceiling of analgesia" characteristic, which means that exceeding the recommended mg/kg dose will not provide increased pain relief. Therefore, if the recommended dose does not relieve pain, the clinician should consider adding an opioid.	Dyspepsia, nausea, vomiting, gastrointestinal bleeding, inhibition of platelet aggregation, acute renal failure, and hepatic toxicity

| Local anesthetics | Lidocaine Bupivacaine EMLA® | Prevents depolarization and blocks the action during the transduction process | Infiltration of surgical incision or wound for peripheral nerve block

Topical application for numbing the skin prior to needle-stick procedures

Component of epidural infusion | Titrate to effect; exceeding recommended dosing can increase risk of systemic toxicity. | Signs of systemic toxicity include nausea, vomiting, tinnitus, blurred vision, hallucinations, weakness, restlessness, anxiety, dizziness, seizures, bradycardia, palpitations, hypotension, apnea, metallic taste, and cardiac arrest.

Topical agents can cause contact dermatitis, burning, and/or edema. |

(continued)

TABLE 3.1 Modified Drug Classification Reference Table From the Children's Hospital Association (*continued*)

Classification	Examples	Mechanism of Action	Indications	Dosage Considerations	Possible Adverse Effects*
Anticonvulsants	Gabapentin Carbamazepine Phenytoin Clonazepam Valproic acid Levetiracetam	Primary indication is not analgesia (additional pain management measures need to be taken). The mechanism of anticonvulsants' effect on pain is believed to be prevention of depolarization and blocking the action potential during the transduction process.	Neuropathic pain	Titrate to relief or intolerable side effects	Adverse effects vary with different anticonvulsants and may also be dose dependent (see Chapter 6, "Coanalgesics" for additional information).

Corticosteroids	Dexamethasone Methylprednisolone Prednisone	Unknown, but may be related to interference with prostaglandin synthesis during the transduction process; shrinkage of tumor mass; tempering of aberrant electrical activity	Neuropathic pain Cancer pain Arthralgia Obstruction pain	A higher dose can be used for acute episodes of severe pain, whereas a lower dose is recommended for chronic, responsive pain.	Associated with administration and withdrawal; risk increases with dose and duration (see Chapter 6, "Coanalgesics" for additional information).

(continued)

Classification	Examples	Mechanism of Action	Indications	Dosage Considerations	Possible Adverse Effects*
NMDA receptor antagonist	Ketamine Methadone	Blocks NMDA receptors at the dorsal horn of the spinal cord during the transmission process. May have other analgesic effects	Neuropathic pain Procedural pain Refractory nociceptive pain	Specific to the actual medication	Nausea, vomiting, drowsiness, sedation, and hallucinations
Alpha2-adrenergic agonists	Clonidine	Not established, (See Chapter 6, "Coanalgesics" for additional information.)	Neuropathic pain	Start with low dose and gradually titrate to relief or intolerable adverse effects	Sedation Hypotension Dry mouth

| GABA agonist | Baclofen Lorazapam Diazepam | Inhibits transmission of monosynaptic and polysynaptic reflexes at the spinal cord during the modulation process | Neuropathic pain Possible acute nociceptive pain | Start with low dose and gradually titrate to relief or intolerable adverse effects | Dizziness Sedation Nausea Constipation with coadministration of opiates; may increase the side effects of dizziness and sedation; withdrawal symptom or seizures if stopped abruptly |

GABA, gamma-aminobutyric acid; NMDA, N-methyl-D-aspartate receptor.

*Note that the potency of opioids varies; when switching from one opioid to another, it is important to utilize an equianalgesic table.

neonate is the lack of study specific to the neonatal population, especially those born prematurely. Most drugs commonly given to neonates are not labeled for use in this population; they are given because they have always been given. A recent study suggests that up to 90% of all medication in the NICU is "off label" (Allegaert, van den Anker, & Naulaers, 2007). Neonates, especially as prematurity increases, are a vulnerable population on which to perform a randomized controlled trial. This off-label drug use does not come without consequences. Research has suggested an increased incidence of kernicterus after widespread use of sulfonamides and of gray baby syndrome from chloramphenicol use in neonates. Despite these experiences, drug therapy in neonates still lacks regular clinical testing and thorough prescribing information (Food and Drug Administration, 2001). Off-label use, although dangerous, is not usually a haphazard use of therapy. It is often a therapy tested through experience and sound judgment in the absence of a controlled trial to use as reference. In 2002, the American Academy of Pediatrics (AAP) Committee on Drugs released a statement on the off-label use of drugs in pediatric patients. The committee stated, "off-label use does not imply an improper use and certainly does not imply an illegal use or a contraindication based on evidence" and "the off-label use of a drug should be based on sound scientific evidence, expert medical judgment, or published literature" (American Academy of Pediatrics Committee on Drugs, 2002).

What we do know is that most drugs will metabolize differently in the neonate and the preterm than in an adult patient. This is because of inherent differences in body surface area, metabolic systems, renal, liver, gut and excretory functions, increased fluid requirement, and concurrent underlying pathologies. These differences become more profound the younger and smaller the neonate.

In the newborn, drug-metabolizing enzymes are immature, particularly CYP2D6 and CYP1A1. CYP3A4 gradually increases with increasing gestational age in preterm infants. The role and substrates of CYP3A7, the fetal form of CYP3A4, remain unknown. In general, phase II or conjugation reactions are inefficient in newborns. They may play an important role in reducing their ability to eliminate xenobiotics. Gastric pH is higher, gastric emptying prolonged, and intestinal absorption is delayed in earlier gestation neonates (Choonara & Conroy, 2002).

Drug distribution is affected by the extreme difference in body composition, especially total fluid and lipid distribution. Differences in developmental expression of metabolic pathways, in addition to immature renal clearance, lead to the profound differences in individual drug biodisposition, especially in very low-birth-weight infants.

In addition to developmental immaturity, these infants may have organ dysfunction related to concomitant disease processes that reduce the clearance or elimination of drugs. This is especially true of hepatic or renal insufficiency. Also, the very measures used to save provide life-saving treatment (e.g., positive pressure ventilation) may reduce hepatic blood flow, which is particularly important for drugs, such as morphine, that have clearance related to hepatic blood flow (Choonara & Conroy, 2002).

A major problem with pharmacology for use in the neonatal population is the limited availability of validated pharmacodynamic endpoints, which are specific testing targets used to see what dosage is safe and effective for this specific population. The situation in neonates is critical because "immaturity of cellular transporters or receptors is likely to alter the effect of drugs, particularly at the low-gestational ages" (Choonara & Conroy, 2002). It is therefore imperative that we are able to see exactly what the effects are for neonates, especially preterms, and not make assumptions based on studies of animals, adults, or even older children. See Box 3.1 for

---

BOX 3.1 What to Consider When Prescribing, Dispensing, and Administering Medications

Time to peak effect

This is the time it takes for patients to experience the maximum effect of the drug. If it does not adequately manage pain by the time of peak effect, it is not effectively relieving the pain.

(continued)

BOX 3.1   What to Consider When Prescribing, Dispensing, and Administering Medications (*continued*)

Half-life

The period of time when half of the pain medication is still left in the circulating serum. Important to know in order to plan for a dosing interval that provides a stable drug effect.

Steady state

Drug administration and drug elimination are equal, providing a steady state of effect. Peak effect and half-life must be considered to reduce peaks and valleys and achieve a steady state.

Metabolites

Metabolism of the medication leads to the formulation of active and inactive metabolites. Active metabolites are the reason for many of the drug's side effects.

Metabolism and excretion

It is important to be aware of the metabolism and excretion rates for medications administered and to decrease the dosage for any patient who has impaired system function, such as with liver failure, kidney failure, gut issues, or prematurity.

Synergy/agonists

The interaction between two medications and a disease process that produces a combined drug effect that is more potent than that achieved by each medication separately.

Counteraction/antagonists

The interaction between two medications and a disease process that produces a combined effect that is less effective than that achieved by each medication separately.

(*continued*)

BOX 3.1   What to Consider When Prescribing,
Dispensing, and Administering Medications (*continued*)

Bioavailability

This refers to the degree and rate at which a medication is absorbed and the percentage of drug that remains unchanged when it reaches the systemic circulation. Bioavailability will be 100% if administered intravenously, but may be reduced if given through a different route that must travel through the circulation.

Distribution

Once the drug is in the systemic circulation, it must then be distributed intercelluarly and interstitially. Drug distribution refers to vascular permeability, regional blood flow, cardiac output, and perfusion rate of the tissue and the ability of the drug to bind tissue and plasma proteins, as well as its lipid solubility. pH also plays a major role in distribution. The drug is easily distributed in the absence of dysfunction in highly perfused organs, such as the liver, heart, and kidneys, and in small quantities through less perfused tissues like muscle, fat, and peripheral organs.

Absorption

Absorption and distribution speak to the same phenomena. *Absorption* is the actual movement of the drug into the blood stream. It is determined by the drug's physicochemical properties, formulation, and route of administration (Le, 2014). If the drug is given intravenously, then absorption is not necessary, the drug is already being directly deposited into the circulation. In addition to the drug's properties, keep in mind the perfusion of the area into which the drug is being introduced (i.e., hypoxia may cause blood shunting away from the gut, which may inhibit or slow the absorbtion of gastrointestinally introduced medications; see Table 3.2 and Figure 3.1).

TABLE 3.2 Some Factors Affecting Drug Absorption Relating to Neonates (Patient Factors Are Particularly Relevant in Neonates)

Physicochemical Factors
Drug formulation
Disintegration of tablets or solid phase
Dissolution of drug in gastric or intestinal fluid
Release from sustained-release preparations
Molecular weight
pK/proportion of drag in ionized/unionized form
Lipid solubility
Patient Factors
General
Surface area available for absorption
Gastrointestinal
Gastric content and gastric emptying
Gastric and duodenal pH
Size of bile-salt pool
Bacterial colonization of lower intestine
Disease states (e.g., short-gut syndrome, biliary atresia)
Muscle
Increased capillary density in neonatal muscle compared with adults increases absorption from muscles

(*continued*)

TABLE 3.2   Some Factors Affecting Drug Absorption Relating to Neonates (Patient Factors Are Particularly Relevant in Neonates) *(continued)*
Reduced cardiac output states reduce absorption
Skin
Blood supply
Peripheral vasodilation
Thickness of skin/stratum corneum
Surface area
Rectal
Rectal venous drainage site
Neonatal absorption > older children

Source: Skinner (2011).

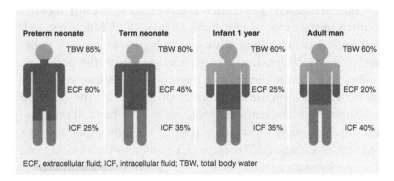

ECF, extracellular fluid; ICF, intracellular fluid; TBW, total body water

FIGURE 3.1. Age-related body water compartments.
Source: Skinner (2011).

important issues to consider about medication selection and administration.

MEDICATION SAFETY

Medication safety is especially important in the preterm and term neonate. These patients have immature body systems— specifically, excretory function, coupled with a smaller mass and service area. This makes dosing particularly difficult. The neonate needs enough of a drug to be effective, but not too much, so as to avoid it building up to a toxic level. In the presence of hypoxemia, blood will be shunted to vital organs and away from the liver, kidneys, and gut. This can lead to impaired functioning of the infant's already immature excretory function.

And there is very limited evidence-based data to know how to safely administer pain medication to these infants. Most drugs given in the NICU are off label and have not been sufficiently tested. Therefore, extreme caution is advised in pharmacological treatment.

An important factor in medication safety is the critical need for safe medication. Medication errors occur as a result of either human mistakes or system flaws (IOM, 2008). Much research has been done, mostly in adults, as to how to ensure safe delivery of drugs. Environment plays a major role in the provider's ability to prescribe the correct therapy, the pharmacist's ability to verify and dispense the correct drug, and for the nurse to administer the medication appropriately. Also, medication delivery involves many individuals so it is a system prone to error (Levine & Cohen, 2007). Table 3.3 reinforces the critical need for checks when administering medication to a patient. Pediatric patients also need to have an accurate weight in order to calculate dosages (as much is weight based). Gestational age of a neonate is also crucial (because of the factors listed earlier in the chapter such as body water percentage).

A 2013 study identified the five recommendations for a safer medication administration system for pediatric nurses:

(a) Implementing the right working environment for medication administration to achieve optimal patient outcomes for medication safety; (b) increasing the level of professional preparation for future pediatric nurses; (c) increasing the level of interdisciplinary communication pertaining to the safe administration of medication to children and their families; (d) standardizing medication delivery and error reporting to promote the safe high-quality delivery of medications for children and their families; and (e) recognizing the unique challenges of pediatric medication delivery and implementing future support for pediatric nurses during the process of medication delivery. (Sears, O'Brien-Pallas, Stevens, & Murphy, 2013, p. 355)

Accurate documentation is critical with all patients, especially neonates. Documentation is not only necessary for legal protection; is a vital communication between disciplines as to what care is planned and administered. Accurate communication prevents errors, which, in this population, can lead to death or lifelong disability.

TABLE 3.3 Eight Rights of Medication Administration
■ Right patient
■ Right drug
■ Right dose
■ Right route
■ Right time
■ Right documentation
■ Right reason
■ Right response

Source: Bonsall (2012).

The use of a computerized, bar-coded medication administration system has also been designed to increase safety with drug administration. These systems typically assign a barcode to each drug and when the barcode is scanned, the information is checked against the medication administration record (MAR). Clinicians also have to scan the patient's identification band as a check that the medication is being given to the right patient. A 2009 NICU study found a 47% reduction in preventable medication errors, adjusted for the number of opportunities for error, through use of a barcoding system (Morriss et al., 2009, pp. 366–367).

REFERENCES

Allegaert, K., van den Anker, J. N., & Naulaers, G. (2007). Determinants of drug metabolism in early neonatal life. *Current Clinical Pharmacology*, 2(1), 23–29.

American Academy of Pediatrics Committee on Drugs. (2002). Uses of drugs not described in the package insert (off-label uses). *Pediatrics, 110*, 181–183.

Bonsall, L. (2012). *Nursing 2012 drug handbook*. Philadelphia, PA: Lippincott Williams & Wilkins and Wolters Kluwer Health.

Choonara, I., & Conroy, S. (2002). Unlicensed and off-label drug use in children: Implications or safety. *Drug Safety, 25,* 1–5.

Food and Drug Administration. (2001). *The Pediatric Exclusivity Provision: January 2001 status report to Congress*. Rockville, MD: Author.

Institute of Medicine. (2008). *Preventing medication errors*. Washington, DC: National Academies Press.

Le, J. (2014). Drug absorption. Retrieved on from www.merckmanuals.com

Levine, S., & Cohen, M. R. (2007). Preventing medication errors in pediatric and neonatal patients. In L. Cohen (Ed.), *Medication errors* (pp. 469–492). Washington, DC: American Pharmacists Association.

Morriss, F. H., Abramowitz, P. W., Nelson, S. P., Milavetz, G., Michael, S. L., Gordon, S. N., . . . Cook, E. F. (2009). Effectiveness of a barcode medication administration system in reducing preventable adverse drug events in a neonatal intensive care unit: A prospective cohort study. *Journal of Pediatrics, 154*(3), 363–368.

Ries, R. K., Fiellin, D. A., Miller, S. C., & Saitz, R. (Eds.). (2009). *Principles of addiction medicine* (4th ed.). Philadelphia, PA: Lippincott Williams & Wilkins.

Sears, K., O'Brien-Pallas, L., Stevens, B., & Murphy, G. (2013). The relationship between work environment and the occurrence of reported paediatric medication administration errors: A pan Canadian study. *Journal of Pediatric Nursing, 28*(4), 351–356.

Skinner, A. (2011). Neonatal pharmacology. *Anaesthesia & Intensive Care Medicine, 12*(3), 79–84.

4

Nonopioids

Nonopioids include any medications that are used for analgesia and are nonnarcotic. Nonopioids can be given alone to manage mild to moderate pain, or may be used in conjunction with an opioid in a coanalgesic manner.

ACETAMINOPHEN

Uses: Mild to moderate pain relief and fever reduction
   Prophylactic use at the time of vaccination is not recommended because of reduced antibody response.

   Oral administration:

      Loading dose 20 to 25 mg/kg

      Maintenance dose 12 to 15 mg/kg/dose

   Rectal suppository:

      Loading dose 30 mg/kg

      Maintenance dose 12 to 18 mg/kg/dose

Note: Rectal administration may lead to toxicity because peak levels may vary widely and may take longer to take effect than oral doses (Birmingham et al., 1997).

   Maintenance intervals: For term infants—every 6 hours

      Preterm equal to or greater than 32 weeks postmenstrual age (PMA)—every 8 hours

      Preterm less than 32 weeks PMA—every 12 hours

Monitoring: Assess for signs and symptoms pain; monitor temperature; assess liver function

Adverse effects: Liver toxicity may occur with excessive doses or therapeutic doses given for more than 48 hours and may lead to symptoms, such as rash, thrombocytopenia, leukopenia, and neutropenia in children.

Pharmacology:

Nonnarcotic analgesia and antipyretic

Peak serum concentration occurs approximately 60 minutes after an oral dose (rectal is variable and prolonged)

Extensively metabolized in the liver, primarily through sulfation with a small amount of glucuronidation; metabolites and any unchanged drug are excreted via the kidneys

Elimination half-life is approximately 3 hours in term neonates, 5 hours in preterm neonates greater than 32 weeks, and up to 11 hours in neonates born earlier than 32 weeks. Elimination is prolonged in patients with liver dysfunction.

Treatment of toxicity: Administration of N-acetylcysteine (NAC) 150 mg/kg in 5% dextrose or one half normal saline (NS) given intravenously (IV) over 60 minutes (loading dose). Followed by 50 mg/kg in 5% dextrose or one half NS over a 4-hour period, then 100 mg/kg in 5% dextrose or one half NS over a period of 16 hours. NAC should be continued until clinical and biochemical markers of hepatic injury improve and acetaminophen concentration is below the limits of detection. NAC solution concentrations of 40 mg/mL have been used to avoid fluid overload and hyponatremia in the neonate (Neofax, 2011).

Acetaminophen is not recommended after immunization in the first months of life as it may blunt the effect of certain immunizations by reducing the body's natural inflammatory response (Prymula et al., 2009).

NONSTEROIDAL ANTI-INFLAMMATORY DRUGS

Nonsteroidal anti-inflammatory drugs (NSAIDs) can be used during infancy. Because of the risk of closure of patent ductus arteriosus (PDA), it is often recommended to wait before administering this drug, especially in a compromised neonate. NSAIDs can offer mild to moderate analgesia and antipyretic effects, with a milder effect on the liver than acetaminophen. Use of NSAIDs has not been studied in preterm infants. Prolonged use of NSAIDs has been linked to renal, circulatory, hepatic, hematological, and gastrointestinal (GI) complications (Anand et al., 2005, 2006).

IBUPROFEN (ADVIL, MOTRIN)

Uses: The bioavailability of ibuprofen is close to 100% and elimination is rapid, even in the presence of liver or renal impairment. Dosage guidelines should be followed as toxicity increases with high doses (Kaufman et al., 1993).

Note: Ibuprofen has only been approved for children older than 6 months of age. Serious risks include GI symptoms such as gastritis, GI bleeding, and acute renal failure.

When possible, calculate ibuprofen dose based on weight using 4 to 10 mg/kg. Give orally every 6 to 8 hours. Maximum single dose is 400 mg/dose, and maximum daily dose is 40 mg/kg/day up to 1,200 mg/day. When weight is unknown, the following guideline based on age may be used (Motrin Prescribing Information, n.d.):

Dose: 4 to 10 mg/kg every 6 to 8 hours

Age 6 to 11 months (weight, 12–17 lb [5.4–8.1 kg])

Dose: 50 mg

Oral drops (50 mg/1.25 mL): 1.25 mL

Age 12 to 23 months (weight, 18–23 lb [8.2–10.8 kg])

Dose: 75 mg

Oral drops (50 mg/1.25 mL): 1.875 mL

LOCAL ANESTHETICS

EMLA (eutectic mixture of local anesthetics) (Neofax, 2011)

Uses: Topical analgesic used for circumcision; not effective for heel lancing.

Topical: 1 to 2 g to distal half of penis, then wrap in occlusive dressing. Allow dressing to remain intact for 60 to 90 minutes. Remove and clean treated area thoroughly prior to circumcision to avoid systemic absorption.

Monitoring: Blood methemoglobin concentration if concerned with toxicity

Adverse effects/precautions: Blanching and redness resolve without treatment. When measured, blood levels of methemoglobin in neonates after application of 1 g of EMLA cream have been well below toxic levels. Two cases of methemoglobinemia in infants occurred after greater than 3 g of EMLA cream was applied; in one of these cases, the infant was also receiving sulfamethoxazole. EMLA cream should not be used in neonates with congenital or idiopathic methemoglobinemia, or who are receiving other drugs known to induce methemoglobinemia, such as sulfonamides, acetaminophen, nitrates, nitroglycerin, phenobarbital, and phenytoin.

Pharmacology: EMLA cream, containing 2.5% lidocaine and 2.3% prilocaine, attenuates the pain response to circumcision when applied 60 to 90 minutes before the procedure. The analgesic effect is limited during the phases associated with extensive tissue trauma such as during lysis of adhesions and tightening of the clamp. EMLA stabilizes the neuronal membranes by inhibiting the ionic fluxes required for conduction and initiation of nerve impulses. There is a theoretic concern about the potential for neonates to develop methemoglobinemia after the application of EMLA cream because a metabolite of prilocaine can oxidize hemoglobin to methemoglobin. Neonates are deficient in methemoglobin nicotinamide adenine dinucleotide (NADH) cytochrome b5 reductase. Lidocaine is metabolized rapidly by the liver to a number of active metabolites and then excreted renally.

Special considerations/preparation: Available in 5-g and 30-g tubes with Tegaderm dressing. Each gram of EMLA contains 25 mg lidocaine and prilocaine 25 mg in a eutectic mixture. pH of the product is 9. It contains no preservatives.

LIDOCAINE

Uses: Topical and/or local anesthetic

Dose: 0.5% to 1% solution (dose should be less than 0.5 mL/kg of 1% lidocaine solution—5 mg/kg)

Bupivacaine, Ropivacaine, Levobupivacaine

Epidural dose: 2.5 mg/kg, one time

Continuous IV infusion: 0.2 mg/kg/hr or less

Liposomal lidocaine 4% cream

REGIONAL BLOCKS

Analgesia can also be administered through a regional block. Some of the main ways it can be given are as a spinal, epidural/caudal, dorsal/penile, or intercostal nerve block. Using this type of analgesia helps to give specific pain relief without the systemic effect (i.e., pain management only where you need it) and does not have the same effect on respiratory status that systemic medication does, such as with opioids (Desborough, 2000).

Spinal block is used for surgical procedures below the umbilicus. There is a risk of inadequate analgesia, incomplete block, or difficulty accessing the site. Caudal or epidural blocks are for surgical procedures of the thorax, abdomen, groin, and lower periphery. There is a risk of inadequate block or improper placement that can lead to nerve damage and/or paralysis. The dorsal penile nerve/ring is used for penile surgery such as hypospadias correction or circumcision. There is a risk of bleeding, and, if epinephrine-containing solutions are used, there is also a risk of end-organ damage (Kraft, 2003). Lastly, there is the intercostal nerve block, which is used for thoracic surgery. There is a risk of pneumothorax with this treatment because of its location to the lungs. With all blocks, only a specially trained, experienced practitioner, such as an anesthesiologist or nurse anesthetist, should insert them.

REFERENCES

Anand, K., Aranda, J., Berde, C., Buckman, S., Capparelli, E., Carlo, W., . . . Walco, G. (2006). Summary proceedings from the neonatal pain-control group. *Pediatrics, 117*, S9–S22.

Anand, K., Johnston, C., Oberlander, T., Taddio, A., Lehr, V. T., & Walco, G. A. (2005). Analgesia and local anesthesia during invasive procedures in the neonate. *Clinical Therapeutics, 27*, 844.

Birmingham, P. K., Tobin, M. J., Henthorn, T. K., Fisher, D. M., Berkelhamer, M. C., Smith, F. A., . . . Coté, C. J. (1997). Twenty-four-hour pharmacokinetics of rectal acetaminophen in children: An old drug with new recommendations. *Anesthesiology, 87*, 244–252.

Desborough, J. (2000). The stress response to trauma and surgery. *Journal of Anesthesia, 85*, 109.

Kaufman, D. W., Kelly, J. P., Sheehan, J. E., Laszio, A., Alfredsson, L., Koff, R. S., & Shapiro, S. (1993). Nonsteroidal anti-inflammatory drug use in relation to major upper gastrointestinal bleeding. *Clinical Pharmacology and Therapeutics, 53*, 485–494.

Kraft, N. (2003). A pictorial guide to circumcision pain. *Advanced Neonatal Care, 3*, 50.

Motrin Prescribing Information. (n.d.). *NcNeil consumer care: Products and dosage.* Retrieved from http://www.motrin.com/product_links/4?val=overview

Prymula, R., Siegrist, C. A., Chlibek, R., Zemlickova, H., Vackova, M, Smetana, J., . . . Schuerman, L. (2009). Effect of prophylactic paracetamol administration at time of vaccination on febrile reactions and antibody responses in children: Two open-label, randomised controlled trials. *Lancet, 374*, 1339–1350.

Opioids

Opioids are a class of drug that promotes decreased pain perception and decreases the reaction to pain; the drug class that includes morphine or morphine sulfate, methadone, and fentanyl or fentanyl citrate. As demonstrated in Figure 5.1, opioids work by binding with specific proteins and opioid receptors found in the brain, spinal cord, gastrointestinal tract, and other organs throughout the body. When the opioid attaches to any one of the receptors, as shown in Figure 5.2, the stimulus of pain to the brain is slowed or blocked, thus reducing the perception of pain. The types of opioids commonly used in neonates include morphine, fentanyl, methadone, and meperidine.

MORPHINE

Morphine and morphine sulfate are similar opioid compounds; morphine sulfate is a salt compound of morphine. Morphine works by stimulating opioid receptors within the posterior amygdala, hypothalamus, thalamus, spinal column, gastrointestinal tract, and the spinal nucleus of the trigeminal nerve. Morphine binds very strongly to the receptor sites, generating an increased sense of pain relief, but also generating a greater sense of sedation and respiratory depression, which contributes to a quicker tolerance and greater dependence. The recommended use for morphine in the neonate is for analgesia, sedation, treatment of opioid withdrawal, and abstinence withdrawal. The recommended dosage is dependent on the purpose or use. Recommendations appear in Table 5.1.

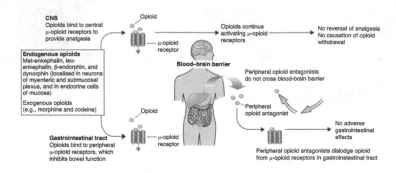

FIGURE 5.1. Path of opioids.

CNS, central nervous system.

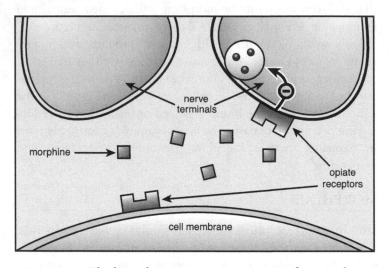

FIGURE 5.2. The brain has many, many receptors for opioids. An overdose occurs when too much of an opioid, such as heroin or oxycodone, fits in too many receptors slowing and then stopping the breathing.

Side effects of morphine include marked respiratory depression, hypotension, bradycardia, ileus and delayed gastric emptying, and urine retention. The receptor sites that morphine has a binding affinity for are found along the dorsal roots innervating the respiratory muscles and gastrointestinal tract, contributing to the relaxation of the smooth muscles

TABLE 5.1 Opioids for Neonates

Name of Drug	Use	Dose and Administration	Adverse Effects	Special Considerations
Fentanyl	Analgesia, sedation, and anesthesia	Sedation/analgesia: 0.5–4 mcg/kg per dose IV slow push Infusion rate: 1–5 mcg/kg/hr Anesthesia: 5–50 mcg/kg	Respiratory depression, chest wall rigidity, and urinary retention	Have Naloxone readily available
Methadone	Treatment of opiate withdrawal	Initial dose: 0.05–0.2 mg/kg every 12–24 hr Reduce dose by 10%–20% per wk over 4–6 wk	Respiratory depression, ileus and delayed gastric emptying, and QT prolongation	Cardiac assessment and careful weaning
Morphine	Analgesia, sedation, treatment of withdrawal	0.05–0.02 mg/kg IV over at least 5 min Continuous infusion: loading dose of 100–150 mcg/kg over 1 hr followed by 10–20 mcg/kg/hr Treatment of opioid dependence: begin at most recent intravenous (IV) morphine dose; taper 10%–20% per day; oral dose is approximately 3–5 times the IV dose Initial treatment of neonatal narcotic withdrawal: 0.03–0.1 mg/kg per dose orally every 3–4 hr; wean dose 10%–20% every 2/3 days	Respiratory depression, abdominal distention, ileus, and urinary retention	Have Naloxone readily available; protect from light

Adapted from Young and Mangum (2009).

of these organs; the side effects are frequently seen after administration. Care must be practiced when administering to provide careful assessment and monitoring to ensure adequate and effective ventilation occurs and is provided if necessary. Frequent monitoring of gastrointestinal function and urine output is necessary.

Withdrawal of morphine must be done carefully and gradually. Tolerance and dependence are common with morphine use and withdrawal must be attempted slowly to avoid central nervous system irritation and seizure activity. Weaning should occur at 10% of original dose once each day as tolerated (Bio, Siu, & Poon, 2011). Discontinuation of medication can be safely done when the infant's dose reaches 0.12 to 0.016 mg/kg/day.

When assessing risks of use in comparison to benefits of use, it is necessary to understand the difference. The risk of use of morphine includes respiratory depression, decreased gastrointestinal motility, and urinary retention, whereas benefits include a deep, effective sedative, and analgesic response for mild to moderate pain. Studies suggest that infants who receive morphine to manage moderate pain tend to require less pain management as adults and are less likely to be resistant to the effects of morphine as adults (Georgia State University, 2008). Studies suggest morphine may have a negative effect on cell life when used without caution or in absence of noxious stimulus (Attarian et al., 2014). Studies also suggest managing neonatal pain appropriately with morphine provides more long-term benefits for healthy neurodevelopmental and adult pain responses than not medicating appropriately.

Limitations of use of morphine when considering the gestational age, weight, and diagnosis of the neonate are controversial and variable. Morphine has a slow onset of analgesic effect—up to 5 minutes, with a peak effectiveness within 15 minutes. Painful procedures or interventions that are emergent should not be managed with morphine. Gestational age considerations focus on organ maturity and enzymatic availability for metabolism. The lower the gestational age, the less mature the neonatal liver—the site of morphine metabolism.

Lower gestational age infants tend to develop tolerance much quicker than their term counterparts, thus creating a need for increasing dosing, which can contribute to increased risk of respiratory depression and hypotension. Use of morphine for management of chronic pain related to mechanical ventilation is controversial as well (Hall & Shbarou, 2009), with use primarily limited to moderate postoperative pain.

FENTANYL AND FENTANYL CITRATE

Fentanyl and fentanyl citrate are synthetic opioids similar in composition to morphine but 50 to 100 times more powerful. Fentanyl citrate is a salt combination of fentanyl and citric acid in a 1:1 mixture. Fentanyl binds to opioid receptor sites in the brain, spinal column, and organs, increasing dopamine release into systemic circulation, thereby generating a sense of relaxation. Fentanyl is also highly lipid soluble, contributing to rebound effects when metabolized from fat cells. Fentanyl use is recommended for analgesia, sedation, and as an anesthetic. The recommended dosage is dependent on the purpose or use. Recommendations appear in Table 5.1.

Side effects of fentanyl include respiratory depression, chest wall rigidity, urinary retention, rapid tolerance with prolonged use, and nausea and vomiting. Care must be taken when administering fentanyl as a slow push to avoid bradycardic episodes. Careful attention to vital signs, urinary output, gastrointestinal function, and respiratory effort is necessary to ensure the infant remains physiologically stable (Taketomo, Hodding, & Kraus, 2001).

Withdrawal of fentanyl must be done judiciously. Fentanyl infusion greater than 2 days will cause negative withdrawal symptoms if infusion is discontinued abruptly. The weaning process is dependent on the length of time the infant received treatment. An infant receiving fentanyl for less than 3 days can reduce the dose by 50% and stop within 24 hours of reduction. An infant receiving treatment for up to 3 to 7 days should receive a dosage reduced by 25% of the maintenance dose every day until the current dose is less than the original dose and then discontinue. Infants receiving fentanyl for greater than 7 days should receive a dose reduced by 10% every 6 to 12 hours as tolerated until the dose is less than original dose, allowing for full discontinuation. The infant's tolerance and stability of vital signs should be closely monitored during the weaning process. Assessment of pain scores will provide guidance for the infant's tolerance and need for adjustment (Taketomo, Hodding, & Kraus, 2001; Young & Mangum, 2009).

Risks and benefits of fentanyl use require the same considerations as the risks and benefits of morphine use. The risk of poor pain management contributes to negative long-term developmental outcomes and more difficult adult pain management. The benefit of neonatal pain management for neurodevelopmental outcomes is important to consider when using fentanyl to manage moderate to severe pain.

When considering the gestational age, weight, and diagnosis of the neonate, fentanyl use has the same limitations and concerns as morphine. Fentanyl has a quick onset of action; a single dose can provide analgesia for procedures. The propensity for fentanyl to cause chest wall rigidity and to depress respiratory function as well as its tendency toward relatively quick tolerance are limitations of the medication. Astute assessment of pain and the use of nonpharmacological methods of pain management are necessary to reduce the need for long-term fentanyl use.

METHADONE

Methadone is a synthetic opioid used for chronic pain associated with opiate withdrawal in neonates. Methadone is a long-acting, protein-binding narcotic. Methadone works similarly to morphine in attaching to opioid receptors in the brain, spinal column, and organs, thereby eliciting a sense of euphoria and blocking pain impulses to the brain. For infants born to mothers who themselves took opioids, such as methadone or street heroin, methadone is a safe, controlled method of managing potential withdrawal pain. Methadone use is recommended for the neonate for treatment and management of opioid withdrawal and abstinence symptoms. The recommended dosage is dependent on its purpose or use. Recommendations appear in Table 5.1.

Side effects of methadone include respiratory depression, ileus, delayed gastric emptying, and potential QT prolongation. Monitoring of respiratory and cardiac function is imperative to avoid adverse outcomes from methadone treatment. Infants born to mothers taking methadone during pregnancy who subsequently experience bradycardia or tachycardia require a 12-lead EKG. Close monitoring of vital signs and prompt intervention for any changes are necessary (Young & Mangum, 2009).

Risks and benefits of methadone use are comparable to morphine and fentanyl; based on the evaluation of the outcomes of the neonate. Evaluation of the maternal history and the potential for neonatal addiction with neurological symptomology is a first step in determining whether to initiate methadone treatment. The benefits of managing the neurological and physiological symptoms of withdrawal far outweigh the negative effects of unsupported withdrawal in the neonate. Risks of cardiac alteration, respiratory depression, and gastrointestinal interruption can be identified and supported through careful and frequent assessment.

When considering the gestational age, weight, and diagnosis of the neonate, limitations of use of methadone focus on the manufacturer's warning of deaths reported during initiation of methadone treatment for opioid dependence. According to the manufacturer, titration that is too rapid without appreciation for the accumulation of methadone over time contributes to respiratory and/or cardiac interruption. Careful and diligent monitoring of vital signs, as well as tightly controlled, strict dosing is imperative to protect the infant.

REFERENCES

Attarian, S., Tran, L. C., Moore, A., Stanton, G., Meyer, E., & Moore, R. P. (2014). The neurodevelopmental impact of neonatal morphine administration. *Brain Sciences, 4*, 321–334. doi:10.3390/brainsci4020321

Bio, L. L., Siu, A., & Poon, C. Y. (2011). Update on the pharmacologic management of neonatal abstinence syndrome. *Journal of Perinatology, 31*(11), 692–701. doi:10.1038/jp.2011.116.Epub2011Aug25

Georgia State University. (2008). Long-term benefits of morphine treatment in infants confirmed in rodent study. *Science Daily.* Retrieved from http://www.sciencedaily.com/releases/2008/11/081103160854.htm

Hall, R. W., & Shbarou, R. M. (2009). Drugs of choice for sedation and analgesia in the NICU. *Clinical Perinatology, 36*(1), 15–26. doi:10.1016/j.clp.2008.09.007

Taketomo, C. K., Hodding, J. H., & Kraus, D. M. (2001). *Pediatric dosage handbook* (8th ed.). Hudson, OH: Lexi-comp.

Young, T. E., & Mangum, B. (2009). *Neofax 2009* (22nd ed.). Montvale, NJ: Thomson Reuters.

Coanalgesics

Coanalgesics, or adjuvant medications, are a group of pharmaceuticals with pharmacological characteristics that were not primarily intended for pain relief but were found to have therapeutic properties when used independently or in conjunction with opioids (Khan, Walsh, & Brito-Dellan, 2011). The list of coanalgesics includes a variety of classes, such as topical medications, anticonvulsants, muscle relaxers, anxiolytics, and sedatives. Specific medications include acetaminophen, nonsteroidal anti-inflammatory drugs (NSAIDs), EMLA, midazolam, dexmedetomidine, phenobarbital, lorazepam, thiopental, chloral hydrate, and lidocaine. Each medication has recommended usages, dosages, side effects, risks, benefits, and limitations based on gestational age, weight, and diagnosis.

Body composition at birth is a special consideration with coanalgesic use. At birth, infants have high body water content in the extracellular space. This, combined with their low body fat and muscle content, this places the infant at higher risk for prolonged duration of action of medications that are redistributed to fat or muscle after first pass (Haidon & Cunliffe, 2010). Renal function is immature at birth, which causes delayed renal drug excretion, contributing to longer half-life of medications. Also contributing to delayed drug excretion and increasing half-life is the immaturity of the liver and the limited availability of liver enzymes. Lastly, the blood–brain barrier is immature at birth, which allows easier passage of medications to the brain, particularly morphine. These considerations are for the term infant; premature infants are at a higher risk because of their decreased physiological capacity to metabolize and excrete medications, therefore, they require more intense monitoring and dosage modifications.

ACETAMINOPHEN

Acetaminophen is an analgesic and an antipyretic used to treat mild pain. The exact mechanism of action of acetaminophen is unknown, but is believed to reduce the level of the inflammatory chemical prostaglandin in the brain.

Acetaminophen helps reduce pain by increasing the pain threshold, which means the pain has to be more severe before the infant actually perceives it. The benefits of using acetaminophen include its ability to reduce pain with nonopioid treatment with little sedative or neurological effects. Side effects of acetaminophen are very rare; however, rash, itch, swelling, thrombocytopenia, leukopenia, and neutropenia have been documented. Close monitoring of vital signs and lab values is necessary if any concerns of side effects exist. Withdrawal of acetaminophen has no contraindications or concerns.

Risks of use of acetaminophen are relative to gestational age, weight, and diagnosis. Infants less than 32 weeks gestation have a longer half-life elimination and require dosing modification. Infants with liver dysfunction have a decreased capacity to metabolize acetaminophen and require dosing modification. Assessment of liver function and consideration of gestational age are necessary before dosing and administration. The recommended use for acetaminophen in the neonate is for mild to moderate pain, especially circumcision pain, and for fever reduction. The recommended dosage is dependent on purpose or use. Recommendations appear in Table 6.1.

NONSTEROIDAL ANTI-INFLAMMATORY DRUGS

NSAIDs are a class of drugs that provide analgesia and antipyretic effects. NSAIDs include aspirin, ibuprofen, and naproxen. NSAIDs work by inhibiting enzymatic development

TABLE 6.1 Coanalgesics for Neonates

Name of Drug	Use	Dose and Administration	Adverse Effects	Special Considerations
Acetaminophen	Antipyretic; mild to moderate pain	Oral loading dose: 20–25 mg/kg Maintenance: 12–15 mg/kg Maintenance intervals: Term: every 6 hr Preterm > 32 wk: every 8 hr Preterm < 32 wk: every 12 hr	Liver toxicity with excessive dosing, rash, fever	
NSAIDs	Mild to moderate pain PDA closure	No current recommendations for pain management	Thrombocytopenia, decreased urine output	
EMLA	Topical analgesia	Apply 1–2 g; cover with occlusive dressing for 60–90 min prior to procedure	Blanching, redness, and methemoglobinemia	
Midazolam	Sedation, anesthesia induction, and refractory seizures	IV: 0.05–0.15 mg/kg **over at least 5 min** Repeat every 2–4 hr PRN Oral: 0.25 mg/kg per dose	Respiratory depression and arrest, hypotension	No rapid infusion

(continued)

TABLE 6.1 Coanalgesics for Neonates (*continued*)

Name of Drug	Use	Dose and Administration	Adverse Effects	Special Considerations
Dexme-detomidine	Sedation	Loading dose: 1 mcg/kg Maintenance: 0.5–0.8 mcg/kg		
Phenobarbital	Anticonvulsant	Loading dose: 20 mg/kg, slowly Maintenance: 3–4 mg/kg per day	Respiratory depression	Close management of IV site
Lorazepam	Anticonvulsant	0.05–0.1 mg/kg	Respiratory depression	Dose dependent CNS depression
Thiopental	Sedation	Up to 2mg/kg; max dose 4 mg/kg		
Lidocaine	Dorsal penile block	Less than 37 wk: 0.5 g Greater than 37 wk: 1 g/kg		Allow at least 5 min for effective pain block before procedure begins

CNS, central nervous system; IV, intravenous; NSAIDs, nonsteroidal anti-inflammatory drugs; PDA, patent ductus arteriosis; PRN, as needed or as the situation arises.

Adapted from Young and Magnum (2009).

of molecules responsible for supporting inflammatory responses in the body. NSAIDs are not typically used in the neonatal population for pain management, although ibuprofen has been used for closure of patent ductus arteriosis. Side effects of NSAIDs include renal dysfunction and interruption of platelets' adhesive properties; these have limited the use of NSAIDs for pain or antipyretic purposes. Although some studies suggest NSAIDs can promote cerebral circulation in neonates, regular use of NSAIDs is still limited.

EMLA

EMLA cream is a topical analgesic containing two anesthetics—lidocaine and prilocaine—in an emulsified cream base. EMLA cream works by releasing analgesic properties of the anesthetics into the epidermal and dermal layers of skin by inhibiting ionic fluxes required for the initiation and conduction of impulses to the brain. The onset, depth, and duration of dermal analgesic effects are dependent on the duration of the application. Once cream is applied to the desired area, an occlusive dressing must be applied. Application of cream should occur at least 1 hour before the procedure for optimal analgesic effect. Analgesic effects can persist for 1 to 2 hours after removal of cream. Risk effects of EMLA cream are the potential for methemoglobinemia from a metabolite of prilocaine that oxidizes hemoglobin into methemoglobin. Caution is needed using EMLA in patients taking sulfonamides, acetaminophen, nitrates, nitroglycerin, nitroprusside, phenobarbital, or phenytoin. Benefits of using EMLA cream as a topical analgesic for circumcision pain far outweigh its risks. The recommended use for EMLA in the neonate is as a topical analgesic for circumcision. The recommended dosage is dependent on purpose or use. Recommendations appear in Table 6.1.

MIDAZOLAM

Midazolam is a benzodiazepine that acts as a sedative, an antiepileptic, and an anesthetic (Pacifici, 2014). Midazolam is short acting with a rapid onset; it is a popular choice of sedation for neonates because of its anxiolytic, muscle relaxant, and anticonvulsant properties. Midazolam is a short-acting medication with a rapid onset of action and a duration of action of 2 to 6 hours. Midazolam has a manufacturer warning for respiratory depression, requiring careful continuous monitoring of respiratory effort in nonintubated patients. Care should be taken not to administer as a rapid bolus infusion. Respiratory depression is attenuated when given in conjunction with opioid narcotics, and care should be taken when using midazolam with patients with central nervous system compromise. Midazolam is effective and provides better sedation for infants when administered with morphine, with no adverse effects. The recommended use for midazolam in the neonate is for sedation, anesthesia induction, and treatment of refractory seizures. The recommended dosage is dependent on purpose or use. Recommendations appear in Table 6.1.

DEXMEDETOMIDINE

Dexmedetomidine or Precedex is a sedative that provides sedation with minimal respiratory depression. Chemically, the actions of dexmedetomidine are similar to clonidine, as it is also an agonist of alpha-adrenergic receptors in the brain. The use of dexmedetomidine is presently off label as a sedative and an analgesic for pediatric patients; studies continue to establish its efficacy and safety (Phan & Nahata, 2008). To date, trials show the use of dexmedetomidine as safe and effective in providing sedation in preterm and full-term infants (Chrysostomou et al., 2013). Dexmedetomidine has shown to be supremely effective in providing safe sedation and analgesia in critically ill, initially intubated, and mechanically ventilated patients. Dosing should be titrated to weight with consideration of gestational age, as studies show neonates have a longer half-life than adults or pediatric patients (Chrysostomou et al., 2013). Risks of use are, thus far, dose dependent without life-threatening adverse effects and the benefit of decreased effect on respiratory effort. Limitations, thus far, focus on the limited use to date in neonates and a need for further studies. Dexmedetomidine is recommended for sedation and analgesia in neonates. The recommended dosage is dependent on purpose or use. Recommendations appear in Table 6.1.

PHENOBARBITAL

Phenobarbital is a long-acting barbiturate drug used primarily for seizure control, that also has good sedative properties. The mechanisms for action in limiting seizure activity are not known, but are believed to involve inhibition of neurotransmission of impulses by enhancing gamma-amino butyric acid (GABA)ergic systems. Phenobarbital has an extremely long half-life of 2 to 7 days. Therapeutic monitoring is necessary even after discontinuation of the medication. Side effects of phenobarbital use include respiratory depression, lethargy, slow feeding, and necrosis after extravasation. Close monitoring of respiratory effort, feeding tolerance, and intravenous (IV) site administration is imperative to reduce negative outcomes of known side effects. The risk-to-benefit ratio shows the benefits of reducing and controlling refractory seizure activity far outweigh the risks of respiratory depression, feeding intolerances, and phlebitis. Close monitoring with careful inspection of the infant throughout treatment will adequately reduce these risks. The recommended use for phenobarbital in the neonate is as an anticonvulsant, although it is still used for its analgesic properties. The recommended dosage is dependent on purpose or use. Recommendations appear in Table 6.1.

LORAZEPAM

Lorazepam is a high-potency benzodiazepine with the ability to reduce anxiety; reduce agitation; treat seizures, nausea, and vomiting; and to relax muscles. Lorazepam is highly protein bound and well distributed through vascular compartments. Onset of action is within 5 minutes and duration of action is 8 to 12 hours in neonates. Lorazepam is typically used as an anticonvulsive when treatment with phenobarbital fails. Risks of use focus solely on its use as a sedative. Lorazepam has been shown to cause myoclonic jerking in premature neonates. Careful observation of IV administration is necessary as lorazepam is caustic to vasculature when extravasation occurs. The recommended use for lorazepam in the neonate is as an anticonvulsant. The recommended dosage is dependent on purpose or use. Recommendations appear in Table 6.1.

THIOPENTAL

Thiopental is a short-acting barbiturate used for anesthetic induction in pediatric patients that is used sparingly in the neonatal population because of its decreased protein binding capacity resulting in higher levels of free drug measurement in the neonate than in the adult (Hall & Shbarou, 2009). The recommended use for thiopental in the neonate is for preintubation or presurgery anesthesia. The recommended dosage is dependent on purpose or use. Recommendations appear in Table 6.1.

LIDOCAINE

Lidocaine is a local anesthetic typically used to manage circumcision pain. Lidocaine works by inhibiting axonal transmission by blocking sodium channels. Although lidocaine is also useful in treating dysrhythmias and seizure activity in neonates, for the purposes of this text, the focus is on its anesthetic properties. Lidocaine is the most widely used local anesthetic for dorsal penile nerve block pain management, with minimal side effects or physiological adverse effects (Taddio, 2001). Risks of use are minimal when compared to benefits of physiological and neurodevelopmental management of pain. Long-term neurodevelopmental changes related to poor pain management support the use of lidocaine as first choice in managing circumcision pain (Taddio, 2001). Side effects include a lingering analgesic effect as long as 4 months in some infants; this lingering effect was identified when observing pain responses to immunizations when comparing circumcised and noncircumcised infants (Hall & Shbarou, 2009). For the purposes of this text, the recommended use for lidocaine in the neonate is for management of circumcision pain. The recommended dosage is dependent on purpose or use. Recommendations appear in Table 6.1.

REFERENCES

Chrysostomou, C., Schulman, S. R., Castellanos, M. H., Cofer, B. E., Mitra, S., Garcia de Rocha, M., . . . Gramlich, L. (2013). A phase II/III, multicenter, safety, efficacy, and pharmacokinetic study of dexmedetomidine in preterm and term neonates. *Journal of Pediatrics, 164*(2), 276–282. doi:10.1016/j.jpeds.2013.10.002

Haidon, J. L., & Cunliffe, M. (2010). Analgesia for neonates. *Continuing Education in Anaesthesia, Critical Care and Pain, 10*(4), 123–127. doi:10.1039/bjaceaccp/mkq016

Hall, R. W., & Shbarou, R. M. (2009). Drugs of choice for sedation and analgesia in the NICU. *Clinical Perinatology, 36*(1), 15–26. doi:10.1016/j.clp.2008.09.007

Khan, M. I., Walsh, D., & Brito-Dellan, N. (2011). Opioid and adjuvant analgesics: Compared and contrasted. *American Journal of Hospital Palliative Care, 28*(5), 378–383. doi:10.1177/1049909111410298

Pacifici, G. M. (2014). Clinical pharmacology of midazolam in neonates and children: Effect of disease—A review. *International Journal of Pediatrics, 2014*, 20. doi:10.1155/2014/309342

Phan, H., & Nahata, M. C. (2008). Clinical uses of dexmedetomidine in pediatric patients. *Paediatric Drugs, 10*(1), 49–69.

Taddio, A. (2001). Pain management for neonatal circumcision. *Paediatric Drugs, 3*(2), 101–111.

Young, T. E., & Mangum, B. (2009). *Neofax 2009* (22nd ed.). Montvale, NJ: Thomson Reuters.

III

Nonpharmacological Management of Acute and Chronic Pain

Nonpharmacological Methods

SUCROSE

Oral sucrose,[1] given 2 minutes prior to a painful procedure, has been shown to decrease heart rate, facial movement, and pain scores in term and preterm infants (Johnson, Stremler, Horton, & Friedman, 1999). Sucrose has been proven to be a safe and effective way to reduce pain from procedures such as a single heel lance and venipuncture (Stevens, Yamada, & Ohlsson, 2004). Optimal pain management of tissue-damaging procedural pain includes the use of sucrose and a pacifier (Fetus and Newborn Committee & Canadian Paediatric Society, 2007). Sucrose may also be beneficial in conjunction with other medication in moderate to severely painful procedures.

SWADDLING/CONTAINMENT/FACILITATED TUCKING

Swaddling is done by wrapping the newborn tightly in a blanket or commercial swaddler to provide containment. Figures 7.1 and 7.2 provide illustrations of both swaddling options.

Containment can also be provided to a preterm baby by using other positioning tools, such as bumpers, bean bags, linen rolls, and so forth, as shown in Figure 7.3. While in utero, the fetus was folded into the amniotic sack with secure, definite boundaries. Allowing an infant's limbs to flail about without the re-creation of such boundaries can cause disorganization and stress, especially in premature infants. During painful situations, the neonate benefits from the comfort of containment,

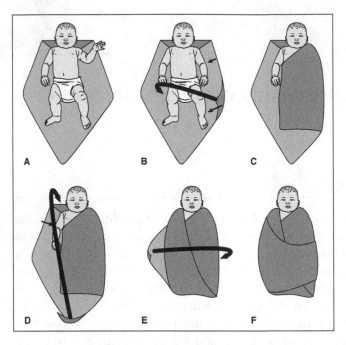

FIGURE 7.1. Facilitated tucking using a blanket and a commercial swaddler.

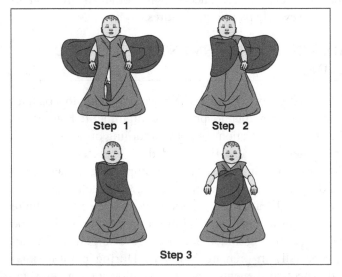

FIGURE 7.2. How to swaddle using a commercial swaddler.

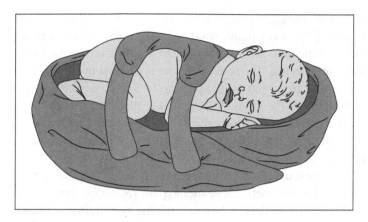

FIGURE 7.3. Facilitated tucking using a positional aid product (such as the Philips "Snuggle Up").

which provides a sense of security. A study of 40 very-low-birth-weight infants showed that facilitated tucking appeared to effectively reduce some of the procedural pain of endotracheal suctioning (Ward-Larson, Horn, & Gosnell, 2004). This is in addition to other research that containment interventions, such as facilitated tucking, may cause significant decreases in the severity of the infant's response to endotracheal suctioning (Evans, 1992; Taquino & Blackburn, 1994).

TOUCH

The power of touch and its healing properties have been utilized for centuries. Recent scientific studies have demonstrated the healing properties of touch. In a study published in 1993, preterm infants experienced a consistent decrease in plasma cortisol levels after massage. Eleven stable infants with a median gestational age of 29 weeks, median birth weight of 980 grams, and median post-natal age of 20 days were studied. Blood samples were obtained to determine levels of adrenaline, noradrenaline, and cortisol 45 minutes before the start of massage and approximately 1 hour after completion of massage. Cortisol, but not catecholamine, con-centrations decreased consistently after massage (median differ-ence –35.8 mmol/L; 95% confidence interval, –0.5 to –94.0;

Wilcoxon matched pairs; Acolet et al., 1993). A more recent study of 59 preterm infants was conducted using Yakson (a Korean touching method) and Gentle Human Touch (a technique used in the United States). The researchers set out to test urine stress hormones and behaviors of infants who had received these healing interventions. The study did not find a quantitative reduction in stress in neonates (through the urine stress hormone levels), but did find an increase in sleep states and a decrease in awake and fussy states (Im & Kim, 2009).

Healing touch, Reiki, and therapeutic touch are among many popular Eastern methods of tactile pain reduction that are used in the adult population, but are gaining recognition for use in neonates.

Other methods, such as craniosacral therapy, chiropractic adjustments, and the Alexander technique, are also new therapies for neonates. Although relatively new, many of these techniques have been around for a long time and have proven successful in adults.

NONNUTRITIVE SUCKING

Sucking is one of a few primitive reflexes that a fetus develops. Its origin is in necessity; the baby needs to suck in order to feed and therefore survive. But the act of sucking without ingesting milk is also soothing to an infant and can be a comfort measure during procedures that cause mild pain (or combined with other measures for more severe pain). It is also a simple and readily available method. Nonnutritive sucking, such as with pacifier or even a gloved finger, can be used during a painful experience to provide a way of coping with pain.

SKIN-TO-SKIN/KANGAROO CARE

Kangaroo care has been around for centuries; research supports this practice, not just for comfort but also to decrease stress caused by pain. In a study published in 2013, 106 healthy, term neonates were randomized to either be held skin to skin or to lay

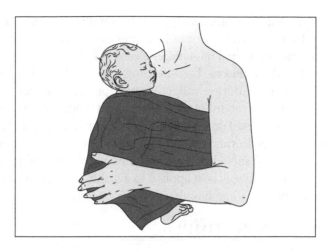

FIGURE 7.4. Skin-to-skin or kangaroo care.

under a radiant warmer during a vitamin K intramuscular injection. Researchers saw a significant reduction in pain response and cry time for the kangaroo group (Abeling & Thacker, 2013). This practice has the benefit of parental empowerment and participation, it facilitates bonding, and causes virtually no risk when the baby is stable. Other studies have produced more modest results. A Cochrane Review published in 2014 that reviewed 19 studies on the effects of skin-to-skin contact showed no significant difference in physiological indicators of pain (in most cases heat rate) but in some cases did show improvement in behavioral indicators (Johnston et al., 2014). This review illustrates the fact that nonpharmacologic methods of pain management do not prevent or decrease pain. Their goal is to decrease stress and anxiety of the neonate so the infant is less affected by the painful stimulus (see Figure 7.4).

BREASTFEEDING

Babies who are feeding orally can benefit from breastfeeding during the painful experience. They will benefit from the soothing sensation of sucking as well as from the natural calming sugar and hormones contained in breast milk. Breastfeeding allows the infant to be pacified through sucking; it provides the warmth and comfort of being next to the mother, along with her familiar rhythmic heart beat and smell; and the breast milk contains oxytocin. Oxytocin is "nature's morphine" and has analgesic properties.

For all of these reasons, breastfeeding is an excellent choice for pain management during mildly painful procedures such as a heel lance. But be careful of the patient's gestational age and oral intake capabilities. For many preterm neonates, particularly before 34 weeks, learning to coordinate feeding may be a stressful endeavor and should not be combined with a painful procedure. This technique is best applied to a stable neonate in whom successful breastfeeding has already been established.

REDUCTION IN STIMULI

Reduction in background stimuli, such as excess light and sound, can help to calm the infant and minimize the stress response to reflect only that of the painful procedure.

MUSIC, SOUND

A 2014 study found that when mothers sang while holding their infants skin-to-skin, it affected the baby's autonomic stability and reduced maternal anxiety (Arnon et al., 2014).

MOVEMENT

Movement, such as rocking and placing baby in a swing, may not be practical during painful procedures. Movement may be a useful distracting tool for babies with chronic pain, colic, painful reflux, and so on. After a painful procedure is completed, movement may help to calm the infant and reduce the stressful reaction.

ACUPUNCTURE/ACUPRESSURE

Acupuncture and acupressure are ancient techniques that have been used to relieve pain for thousands of years in China and other areas of the world. Acupuncture is the placement of tiny needles at particular channels or points throughout the body (acupressure is the application of pressure to these same areas).

Many scientific studies have been done recently on the efficacy of such therapies, but few have been conducted on the neonatal population. In a study published in 2010, 97 neonatal intensive care unit (NICU) patients who had a perinatal brain injury were enrolled in a controlled trial with acupuncture. The results showed that with combined acupuncture and rehabilitation, the infants had improved mental and physical development when followed until 34 months of age (Cao, Hu, & Tan, 2010). Another retrospective study aimed at showing the feasibility, safety, and potential therapeutic effects in inpatient infants was conducted in 2011 in the hope of minimizing the amount of sedative and analgesic drugs babies were exposed to (Gentry, McGinn, Kundu, & Lynn, 2012). Although there were no strong causal findings, acupuncture did show resolution of chronic agitation and feeding issues in some of the babies. The study also found that acupuncture was well tolerated and feasible even in an intensive care setting (Gentryet al., 2012).

NOTE

1. For the purposes of this book we are not considering sucrose a drug. There is debate over whether it should be considered a medication or a nonpharmacological method of treatment. Please use necessary precautions with all treatment methods and monitor the patient closely.

REFERENCES

Abeling, B. A., & Thacker, A. D. (2013). The impact of kangaroo care on pain in term newborns receiving intramuscular injections. *Journal of Obstetric, Gynecologic, & Neonatal Nursing, 42,* S89. doi:10.1111/1552-6909.12182

Acolet, D., Modi, N., Giannakoulopoulos, X., Bond, C., Weg, W., Clow, A., & Glover, V. (1993). Changes in plasma cortisol and catecholamine concentrations in response to massage in preterm infants. *Archives of Disease in Childhood, 68,* 29–31.

Arnon, S., Diamant, C., Bauer, S., Regev, R., Sirota, G., & Litmanovitz, I. (2014). Maternal singing during kangaroo care led to autonomic stability in preterm infants and reduced maternal anxiety. *Acta Paediatrica, 103,* 1039–1044. doi:10.1111/apa.12744

Cao, W., Hu, M., & Tan, L. (2010). Effect of combined acupuncture and rehabilitation on high-risk infants with perinatal brain injuries. *Journal of Acupuncture and Tuina Science*, 8(4), 222–225. doi:10.1007/s11726-010-0412-1

Evans, J. C. (1992). Reducing hypoxemia, bradycardia, and apnea associated with suctioning in low birthweight infants. *Journal of Perinatology*, 12, 137–142.

Fetus and Newborn Committee, & Canadian Paediatric Society. A Joint Statement with the American Academy of Pediatrics and the Fetus and Newborn Committee, Canadian Paediatric Society. (2007). Prevention and management of pain in the neonate: An update. *Paediatrics & Child Health*, 12(2), 137–138.

Gentry, K. R., McGinn, K. L., Kundu, A., & Lynn, A. M. (2012). Acupuncture therapy for infants: A preliminary report on reasons for consultation, feasibility, and tolerability. *Pediatric Anesthesia*, 22, 690–695. doi:10.1111/j.1460-9592.2011.03743.x

Im, H., & Kim, E. (2009). Effect of Yakson and Gentle Human Touch versus usual care on urine stress hormones and behaviors in preterm infants: A quasi-experimental study. *International Journal of Nursing Studies*, 46(4), 450–458.

Johnson, C. C., Stremler, R., Horton, L., & Friedman, A. (1999). Effect of repeated doses of sucrose during heel stick procedure in preterm neonates. *Biology of the Neonate*, 75, 160–166.

Johnston, C., Campbell-Yeo, M., Fernandes, A., Inglis, D., Streiner, D., & Zee R. (2014). Skin-to-skin care for procedural pain in neonates. *Cochrane Database of Systematic Reviews*, 1, CD008435. doi:10.1002/14651858.CD008435.pub2

Stevens, B., Yamada, J., & Ohlsson, A. (2004). Sucrose for analgesia in newborn infants undergoing painful procedures. *The Cochrane Database of Systematic Reviews*, 3, CD001069.

Taquino, L., & Blackburn, S. (1994). The effects of containment during suctioning and heelstick on physiological and behavioral responses of preterm infants. *Neonatal Network*, 13(7), 5.

Ward-Larson, C., Horn, R., & Gosnell, F. (2004). The efficacy of facilitated tucking for relieving procedural pain of endotracheal suctioning in very low birthweight infants. *American Journal of Maternal Child Nursing*, 29(3), 151–156.

Developmental Considerations

Developmental considerations are imperative in delivering comprehensive and safe care to neonates in the neonatal intensive care unit (NICU). Developmental considerations are not only necessary when assessing and supporting physiological function, growth, and musculoskeletal growth, but also affect normal neurological outcomes and pain mitigation. The lower the gestational age of the infant, the more fragile its neurological status when considering brain maturity and neurological innervation. Prevention of aberrant neuronal pathways is crucial in ensuring productive and positive outcomes for all neonates born at any gestational age. Much research detailing the short- and long-term sequelae resulting from disruption of normal neuronal development of neonates is available (Evans, 2001; Grunau, 2013; Grunau, Holsti, & Peters, 2006). Promoting health care team behaviors and interventions that reduce the negative stimuli and support the infant through unavoidable stimuli are known to promote positive outcomes. Developing such methods of care is necessary for all health care workers and for families.

Neonates are exposed to upward of 74 painful experiences per 24-hour period. This number increases with decreasing gestational age, with a 24-week gestation infant potentially experiencing upward of 150 painful experiences, namely separation from his or her mother, per 24-hour period. Neurological development continues along a prescribed continuum, whether in utero or born prematurely, with neuronal synaptic connections and myelination of those neurons incomplete until almost the fifth birthday. Infants born between 23 and 34 weeks are at greatest risk for rewiring of the normal pathways that establish appropriate responses to stimuli. Interfering with the development of recognition and response to painful stimuli can have short- and long-term effects that alter the infant for life (Grunau, 2013).

The brain develops in five stages, beginning with proliferation during the first 8 to 16 weeks of gestation, and continuing through myelination, which occurs through adulthood (Kenner & Lott, 2003). Proliferation begins with the production of neurons and glial cells, which protect and nourish the neurons while guiding the correct migration of neural cells. Migration occurs during 12 to 20 weeks gestation, when neurons begin migration into the cerebral cortex to differentiate. Synaptogenesis begins at 8 weeks gestation and is the process of making connections between neuronal cells during proliferation and migration for organization into specific functions. Organization begins at around 24 weeks and continues through adulthood. During this stage, experiential input and environmental influences will increase or decrease the synaptic connections while glial cells increase in number to nourish the developing neuronal cells. The organization stage is a period for hardwiring specialized function and action of neuronal cells. The final stage, myelination, begins around 24 weeks gestation and continues through adulthood. During the myelination stage, the neuronal cells are covered with a lipoprotein shell that helps facilitate conduction of neuronal impulses (Kenner & Lott, 2003).

All experiential stimulus and environmental influences have great potential to alter the future machinations of the neuromuscular and neurodevelopmental status of the infant. Negative stimulus, pain stimulus, prolonged exposure to noxious stimuli, and lack of positive feedback can all alter the hardwiring of the neuronal organization of the brain. Consideration of the simultaneous development of the sensory system with brain development generates a sense of urgency in clinicians who are striving to understand the impact of environment on developmental outcomes of fragile neonates.

The sensory system develops in a sequential, orderly manner regardless of gestational age at birth. Development and maturity will continue at the programmed rate and stage, with life in the extrauterine environment only having a negative effect if the infant is not well protected. The tactile system develops first, as early as 8 weeks gestation, and is fully functional by 12 weeks. The tactile system is most mature and most sensitive in the feet, hands, and perioral tissue creating a conundrum for health care workers rendering care for premature infants (Kenner & Lott, 2003). Much negative stimulus centers on the feet for heel sticks for blood sampling and the perioral area for intubation and orogastric tube insertion.

Next is the vestibular system, which is functional by 10 to 14 weeks. The gustatory and olfactory senses develop next, with the auditory system not being complete until 19 to 25 weeks. The visual system develops last, with full maturity not achieved until the end of 1 postnatal year. The visual system begins development around 20 weeks gestation, but does not reach functioning capacity until 38 weeks gestation when the fetus remains in utero. Acceleration of functional units of the visual system is only appreciable for opening of the fused lids and capacity to send stimuli responses to the brain. Focusing, pupillary constriction, and visual acuity do not accelerate in the absence of the uterus (Grunau et al., 2006).

With a basic understanding of the sequence of brain development comes a deeper understanding of how environmental stressors and stimuli can alter that normal process. A myriad of considerations is necessary when approaching assessment care, social interactions, and medical interventions of the fragile neonate to ensure protection of fragile and growing neurological systems to support optimal outcomes. Any alteration in normal sequential development becomes a negative, unpleasant sensory experience for the infant, contributing to increasing risks for pain and thus requiring knowledge of management of that pain.

The short-term impact of pain and stress in the neonate repeatedly exposed to routine care and procedures in the NICU include peripheral, spinal cord and supraspinal processing neuroendocrine functions, and neurological development (Whit-Hall & Anand, 2005). Alterations in physiological stability, such as desaturations and bradycardic episodes, are common in infants experiencing pain. The developmental impact for unmanaged pain can last a lifetime while creating immediate care interventions.

The long-term impacts of pain and stress in the neonate include permanent and abnormal pain thresholds, increased incidence of anxiety disorders, attention deficit disorders, and/or exaggerated startle reflexes, to name a few (Whit-Hall & Anand, 2005). Altering the neuronal pathways early in life will create a brain that responds to pain stimuli differently and abnormally. Delayed pain responses or no neurological recognition of pain creates a scenario that can put the infant at risk for life. Inability to recognize or respond to pain will put the infant at risk for future potentially catastrophic injury, such as foot injuries with severe infections if diabetes develops. Increased incidences of anxiety disorders have been documented in children who were born prior to 34 weeks and parental report of limited management of pain during daily activities in the NICU (Whit-Hall & Anand, 2005). These alterations and abnormal neurological development can affect neuromuscular development, meeting developmental milestones, and leading fully productive lives as adults.

Developmental positioning and pain management practices for all infants regardless of gestational age must focus on promoting rest and sleep above all. Providing containment holding during and after procedures or treatments, reducing unnecessary stimulus through cluster care, and promoting the inclusion of families in the care team help ensure sleep remains as uninterrupted as possible. Promoting cue-based care for assessments and feedings allows the infant to guide the interactions. Understanding and respecting the sleep and behavior states when planning procedures, interventions, and interactions for the infant helps ensure the infant is ready for our needs. The ultimate goal is providing an environment that mimics the uterine environment as closely as possible to promote the best neurological development and outcomes possible, with more caution and attention paid to the needs of infants with decreasing gestational age.

Developmental positioning and pain management practices by gestational age beginning at 24 to 28 weeks should focus on promoting sleep and rest as a priority, through clustered care, reducing effects of gravity, and environmental manipulation. Providing boundaries and swaddling to promote midline orientation and flexion will promote normal neuromuscular development. Limiting light exposure, controlling for noise exposure, and protecting skin hydration and fluid balance with proper hydration and humidity all work to support midline orientation, neurological development, and recreation of the uterine environment. The goal is always to put the infant back in the uterus in our world as best or as close as we can. Gravity is a force working against supporting musculoskeletal development and alleviating pain. Pain management practices should make the reduction of stressors and interventions a priority. Clustering care, encouraging parents to participate in skin-to-skin practices, providing colostrum oral care, and limiting environmental stressors will reduce the negative experiences, thus reducing the exposure to pain (Kenner & McGrath, 2004). Supportive use of positioning tools, such as soft blanket rolls, that provide boundaries and containment but not barriers—remember, the uterus was flexible—and use of foam, gel, and cushions as available to mitigate the effects of gravity are imperative for this gestational age. Positioning aids to promote neutral head alignment for the first 48 to 72 hours; boundaries provide containment of feet, flexion of shoulders and hips, and encourage hand-to-mouth movement even if intubated—all help to recreate the womb. Use of sucrose and pharmacological options for more invasive or prolonged interventions are necessary considerations to promote optimal outcomes at this gestational age.

Developmental positioning and pain management practices by gestational age beginning at 27 to 31 weeks should focus on continuing to control for light and noise, while working to reduce external stimuli and limit the effects of gravity. Continue to use positioning aids to promote neutral alignment to promote midline orientation, rounding hips and shoulders; promoting physiological flexion is imperative as this is the organizational stage of neuronal development. Promoting normal organization and hardwiring ensures limiting sequelae of negative stimulus and influences. Containment, midline orientation, flexion of shoulders and hips, and comfort are paramount during this developmental stage of growth. Use of positioning aids, limiting sound and light stimulus, and clustering care are imperative. Education of the families continues to focus on appropriate handling, interactions, and encouraging bonding in developmentally appropriate ways.

Developmental positioning and pain management practices by gestational age beginning at 32 to 35 weeks begin with focusing on integrating the neonate into the extrauterine environment with gentle introduction to the nursery environment. Transitioning to open cribs and thus more sound and light exposure creates a challenge for the clinician. Practicing cyclic lighting to promote the establishment of circadian rhythm and limiting light exposure to daylight hours will help habituate the infant to day–night rhythms. Continuing to provide boundaries through swaddling supports organization and myelination of synaptic connections for smooth state transitions (Kenner & McGrath, 2004). Bottle feeding and suckling at the breast may be introduced at this gestational age—stimulus that should be a pleasant nutritive experience for the infant and a positive bonding experience for the mother. Encouraging these types of positive interactions with the parents are important to establish the positive hardwiring of pleasant stimulus and interactions.

Developmental positioning and pain management practices by gestational age beginning at 34 to 40 weeks consider the range of ages; the infant closer to 34 weeks will still require supportive and protective consideration of visual development. Light protection continues to be a focus during this gestational age for fragile and underdeveloped visual structures. Noise is also a consideration and, although the older infant closer to 40 weeks will be better able to process noise stimulus, supporting a quieter environment is still necessary to improve myelination and continue synaptic development for appropriate processing. As the infant gets closer to the 40-week gestational age—actual or corrected—less consideration to proliferation of neuronal cells is necessary, but a focus on supporting correct neurodevelopmental organization is still paramount.

Developmental positioning approaches not only facilitate pain management and comfort but also promote appropriate neurological development to reduce long-term sequelae. Each positioning approach carries its own impact, beginning with hands to mouth, and incorporating several others.

Facilitated tuck is a method of positioning using positioning aids or hands that promote hand-to-mouth behavior, calming, and nonpharmacological pain management. Placing hands on the neonate's head, and holding feet and legs to the stomach promotes midline orientation and provides boundaries for containment. Facilitated tuck is also known as hand swaddling (Figure 8.1).

Boundaries, such as blanket rolls and commercial containment products, provide the neonate with the artificial uterine environment that promotes midline orientation and hand-to-mouth behaviors. The use of soft blanket rolls, without regard to gestational age, promotes the alignment and shaping of the musculoskeletal system that occurs naturally in the uterus. Effective boundaries promote flexion and midline orientation. Boundaries created through swaddling offer warmth, reduce extraneous movement, promote developmental flexor tone, and support neuromuscular development, which can also be an adjunct pain management intervention (Kenner & McGrath, 2004). Boundaries are an important treatment modality for promoting appropriate neuromuscular and neurodevelopmental outcomes. Through appropriate re-creation of the uterine

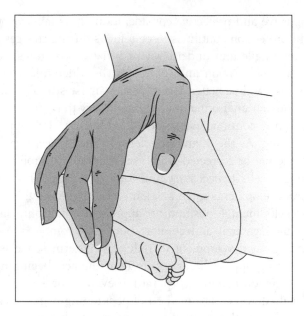

FIGURE 8.1. Infant in facilitated tuck.

environment, supportive sequential development can occur, which works to offset the hostile clinical environment in which the infant is surviving during the first weeks of life (Figure 8.2).

Prone positioning provides many medical and developmental advantages. The medical advantages include better oxygenation and ventilation, better gastric emptying, reduced reflux, decreased risk of aspiration, less energy expenditure, better sleep and less crying, and less sleep apnea (Kenner & McGrath, 2004). The developmental benefits of prone positioning include facilitating development of flexor tone, hand-to-mouth activities, active neck extension, head raising, and forearm propping; coping mechanisms are also improved. Prone positioning does interfere with socialization of the infant because it decreases the ability to make eye contact. The medical and developmental benefits transcend the gestational ages—the benefits are realized from 23 to 43 weeks (Figure 8.3).

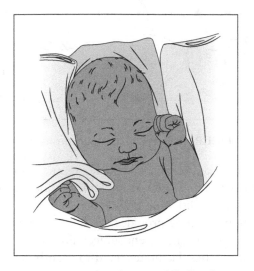

FIGURE 8.2. Infant swaddled with
blanket boundaries.

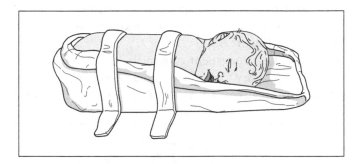

FIGURE 8.3. Infant in prone position.

The advantages of supine positioning include easier access
for medical care, a reduction of sudden infant death syndrome
(SIDS) in term infants, easier visual exploration for the infant,
and the facilitation of socialization. Supine positioning can help
reduce lateral head flattening caused by side-lying positioning,

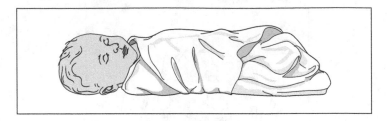

FIGURE 8.4. Infant in supine position.

but has been linked to brachycephaly. Supine positioning can encourage extension of head, neck, and shoulders and must be considered when positioning (Figure 8.4).

Side-lying positioning provides better gastric emptying than a prone or supine position, encourages midline orientation of head and extremities, facilitates hand-to-mouth behaviors, and counteracts external rotation of limbs (Kenneth & McGrath, 2004). Side lying can help reduce symptoms of a number of lung disease by contributing to better oxygenation. Side lying requires assuring that shoulders are rounded; the top hip and shoulder remain slightly forward to reduce the weight bearing of the lower hip (Figure 8.5).

Developmentally congruent care in the NICU, in a nursery, or at home is necessary to ensure optimal neurological outcomes and zero pain. Abating pain is a paramount concern as well.

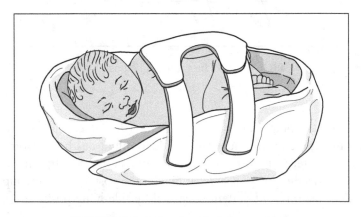

FIGURE 8.5. Infant in side-lying position.

When integrating principles of developmentally relevant care with gestational age considerations, optimal outcomes can be expected and pain can be controlled or eliminated. Pain as a response to inappropriately overstimulated sensory experiences can be managed and reduced when following the established guidelines for developmentally appropriate care in any particular unit. Reducing noxious stimuli and promoting positioning and flexion are crucial in establishing protocols to champion developmentally appropriate and sound care.

REFERENCES

Evans, J. C. (2001). Physiology of acute pain in preterm infants. *Newborn and Infant Nursing Reviews, 1*(2), 75–84. doi:10.1053/nbin.2001.25302

Grunau, R. E. (2013). Neonatal pain in very premature infants: Long-term effects on brain neurodevelopment, and pain reactivity. *Rambam Maimonides Medical Journal, 4*(4), e0025. doi:10.5041/RMMJ.10132

Grunau, R. E., Holsti, L., & Peters, J. W. (2006). Long term consequences of pain in human neonates. *Seminars in Fetal and Neonatal Medicine, 11*, 268–275.

Kenner, C., & Lott, J. W. (2003). *Comprehensive neonatal nursing: A physiological perspective* (3rd ed.). St. Louis, MO: Saunders.

Kenner, C., & McGrath, J. (2004). *Developmental care of newborns and infants: A guide for health professionals.* St. Louis, MO: Mosby.

Whit-Hall, R., & Anand, M. B. (2005). Short- and long-term impact of neonatal pain and stress: More than an ouchie. *NeoReviews, 6*(2), e69–e75. doi:10.1542/neo.6-2-e69

IV

Integration of Treatment Methods

Multidisciplinary Approach

A multidisciplinary approach that includes the physician, registered nurse, physician assistant, advanced practice nurse, and, most important, the family members is imperative in providing comprehensive pain management for all infants. Consideration of the role of each team member in mitigating infant pain and providing comfort, as well as promoting communication among members of the team is fundamental to the best interests of the infants. Each member of the team has a unique perspective and bears responsibility for recognizing and providing interventions for recognized pain. Providing techniques for communicating those responsibilities becomes the challenge. First, identification of each individual's role and responsibility is necessary before communication techniques can be discussed.

MEDICAL APPROACH

Physicians, neonatologists, and pediatricians, including medical residents in pediatric rotation, have an obligation and responsibility for the medical management of the infant, whether in a newborn nursery or a neonatal intensive care unit (NICU). The primary responsibility is the medical management of physiological function and disease management. Directives for physiological management in the form of written or electronic orders directing the interventions are given by the physician team. Ideally, the physician should conduct a comprehensive head-to-toe assessment and have a first hand understanding and working knowledge of the physiological condition of the patient. The key role of the physician in mitigating neonatal pain is detection and management of the pain (Boyle & McIntosh, 2004).

Likewise, the roles of the physician assistant and advanced practice nurse are similar to that of the physician. Primary responsibility for the medical management of physiological stability of the infant falls to the physician assistant and advanced practice nurse. Each is also responsible for providing written or electronic orders for interventions that provide physiological stability and direct the support team's activities and interventions.

NURSING APPROACH

The registered nurse has the primary responsibility of assessing physiological systems and the effects of interventions and treatments, administering and monitoring medications, and educating families. Comprehensive head-to-toe assessments are necessary to monitor the effects of interventions. Written or electronic documentation of findings is also a necessary responsibility. The registered nurse's primary role in mitigating neonatal pain is recognizing, appropriately assessing, reporting the findings, administering and managing nonpharmacological and pharmacological interventions, and assessing the effects of those interventions.

FAMILY APPROACH

The family's role is to provide support for and advocate for the newborn. Unable to verbalize concerns or needs independently, the neonate is dependent on the family to provide his or her voice. The family has a responsibility to the infant to ensure adequate and safe care is rendered, while providing a voice when further support may be necessary. The family can be key to identifying and reporting pain to health care workers and, as such, are an integral part of the team (Friedrichs, Young, Gallagher, Keller, & Kimura, 1995). The role of the family in mitigating neonatal pain is to understand pain cues of the infant and report and advocate for interventions to treat the pain.

COMMUNICATION IS KEY

A key responsibility in the role of each member of the team is communication. Each member of the team has a responsibility to the neonate to collaborate and communicate, with the infant the primary focus of the interaction. All too often, breakdown in communication between one or more member of the team leads to misunderstanding and, for the purpose of pain management, leaves an infant without adequate support. It is fundamentally imperative for each member of the team not only to understand each other's role, but to find a way to communicate effectively. A recent position statement set forth by pain management task forces formed through neonatal and pediatric organizations suggests a multidisciplinary approach is necessary for all nonverbal patients (Herr et al., 2006). The National Association of Neonatal Nurses provides a guideline for pain assessment and management of neonates and directs health care workers to take a collaborative and interdisciplinary approach to identifying and managing neonatal pain (Walden & Gibbins, 2008; Figure 9.1).

Methods that can promote effective communication include education, case studies, debriefing, and pain committees.

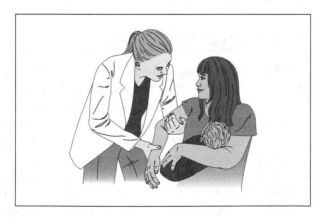

FIGURE 9.1. Families should communicate with the health care team members.

Education of both health care workers and family members is essential in management of neonatal pain. Walden and Gibbins (2008) suggest all nurses working in NICUs should receive education and competency validation in pain assessment and management skills upon hire and periodically throughout employment. At a minimum, the education should include the anatomy and physiology of pain transmission, modulation, and perception and the physiological and behavioral indicators of pain. Education of pain management for the registered nurse should include nonpharmacological approaches, pharmacological interventions, special procedural techniques, and end-of-life pain management (Walden & Gibbins, 2008). Educational opportunities should also include instruction on how to identify differences in pain for gestational ages and developmental stages. A competent understanding of safe medication administration and adverse effects of pharmaceuticals is necessary. Education should also include the ability to educate the family on pain assessment and management as appropriate for their involvement. The education should include appropriate documentation of pain-assessment findings and intervention responses. Finally, education should include the ability to communicate appropriately with the interdisciplinary team regarding the assessment and intervention status of the infant (Walden & Gibbins, 2008).

HOW TO IMPROVE EDUCATION

Education of the physician team should focus on the physiological and behavioral cues of the infant by gestational and developmental stages. A focus on an understanding of the underlying factors that can alter the infant's ability to demonstrate pain symptoms should be part of the education as well. A focus on the long-term effects of poor pain management will be useful for physicians in understanding the need for pain management at all gestational ages for all painful interventions (Schultz, Loughran-Fowlds, & Spence, 2009). An educational focus on assessment, appropriate interventions, and postintervention assessment are necessary elements. Communication techniques with the family and interdisciplinary team are a focus for education and annual competency as well.

CASE STUDIES AS LEARNING TOOLS

Case studies are a great tool for interdisciplinary collaboration and learning. Using case studies of current, past, or fictional patients is a nonthreatening, informal method of bringing team members together to review symptoms, interventions, and outcomes of pain management. Case studies promote teamwork and communication skills (Bradshaw & Lowenstein, 2014). The Institute of Medicine (IOM) recommends interdisciplinary systematic reviews of practice guidelines and patient outcomes in an effort to promote quality improvement and improving patient outcomes (Newhouse & Spring, 2010). Case studies promote critical thinking, problem-solving, and decision-making skills of health care workers, which aligns with the IOM recommendation for promoting quality improvement. Systematic review of events presented during a case study can foster communication about what is known about the patient, what is understood about the patient, and where gaps in that knowing and understanding exist.

Elements of a case study for promoting critical thinking, problem-solving, and decision-making skills, as well as communication skills include the problem or situation, the patient scenario, each participant's contribution, priorities and a solution, implementation of the solution, and results. Presentation of the problem or situation will provide the situation, background, and assessment of the scenario in a neutral format, without consideration of discipline or outcome. It requires simple, straightforward, unbiased accounting of the events and circumstances. Next, each discipline's contribution to the recommendations and outcomes can be presented and reviewed, ideally without opinion or commentary from other disciplines. Remaining neutral when reporting facts will promote collaboration without creating barriers or placing responsibilities on a particular discipline. Keeping information strictly factual is key.

Once all salient information is presented and understood by all members present, a group discussion of what each discipline deems a priority can ensue. A word of caution: It may be wise to include a nonbiased, third party to ensure discussions remain productive and not accusatory, as the intent is to promote quality, not point blame, especially when reviewing particularly difficult cases. Ideally, to build communication skills, a team new to case study activities should begin with patient outcomes that were positive.

Once priorities from each discipline are determined, a discussion can begin about the rationale for the priority with recommendations for a solution. The recommendations should be supported with evidence-based research and documented proof of outcomes, not simply based on practitioner comfort or experience. Using the IOM recommendation of promoting outcomes through evidence-based research is key in promoting best practices and establishing consistent standards of care. Comparison of interventions that were implemented to evidence-based research can be the key to overcoming barriers, communication gaps, and advancing practice to the standards supported by evidence. Review of the implemented interventions and the response and outcomes can provide robust conversation for improving processes for future patients. Identifying the gaps in knowledge from any contributing discipline and working collaboratively to overcome those gaps not only improves patient outcomes, but also works to promote teamwork and communication.

Case studies are a useful and productive tool for promoting critical thinking skills and communication retrospectively in a controlled, planned atmosphere. Debriefing allows a similar process to take place in a more abbreviated format in a more real-time manner. Debriefing is a conversation between care providers that includes the sharing and examination of information after a specific event takes place. The Agency for Healthcare Research and Quality (AHRQ) provides comprehensive tools and support to promote health care communication that promotes patient safety in response to the IOM reports of improving patient outcomes. Debriefing is a tool AHRQ provides through the TeamSTEPPS initiative—an evidence-based program with the singular goal of promoting patient safety (AHRQ, n.d.).

DEBRIEFING

The debriefing checklist created by the AHRQ through the TeamSTEPPS initiative covers nine elements of review. This systematic, organized review should include all persons intimately involved in the situation for review, including parents. The elements of the debriefing tool cover communication concerns, task assistance, resources, and process-improvement elements of what went well and what needs adjustment. Using the debriefing tools when considering managing neonatal pain is a productive way to include all members of the team.

A debriefing session can occur after each episode of neonatal pain, with review of the nine elements to promote a better outcome for future episodes of pain. Include all team members in the review to determine whether communication was clear: Did everyone understand his or her roles and responsibilities in alleviating pain? Were the resources available to alleviate the pain, and, if so, were they successful? Should anything change for the next episode? Debriefing is simple, comprehensive, and timely in promoting patient outcomes. Debriefing can be highly effective in engaging all members of the team, promoting communication skills in an objective manner, and focusing on the patient.

DEBRIEFING CHECKLIST

The team should address the following questions during a debriefing:

___ Was communication clear?
___ Were roles and responsibilities understood?
___ Was situation awareness maintained?
___ Was workload distribution equitable?
___ Was task assistance requested or offered?

____ Were errors made or avoided?
____ Were resources available?
____ What went well?
____ What should improve?

Adapted from the AHRQ website.

PAIN COMMITTEE APPROACH

Pain committees are another method used to promote interdisciplinary collaboration and to align with IOM recommendations, while focusing on patient outcomes. Pain committees should include one member of each disciplinary team responsible for mitigating neonatal pain—physicians, advanced practice nurses, registered nurses, pharmacists, and families. Each member should have an equal say in the development of an individualized pain management plan. Each member of the team has valuable insight and experience to contribute. Pain committees should meet at regular intervals. Although the pain committee will contribute to the development of individualized pain management plans for neonates, the pain committee should also have activities that are more global.

As a committee, each member should have a working knowledge of the pain management policies and philosophy of the organization. The committee should have the responsibility for developing, implementing, and maintaining currency of all pain management policies that drive patient management. The committee should have a method and process for communicating the policies to all new families and employees. Once a comprehensive policy and a method for communicating the language of that policy are in place, the committee can work to develop its goals.

The goals of a pain committee should include assurance that the committee's objectives align with the organizational vision and mission; the committee must have a process in place for systematic review of objectives and outcomes. Committee objectives that align with organizational visions ensure organizational support and encourage compliance from all members in adhering to the principals set forth by the committee. Systematic review processes ensure performance improvement is an ongoing process, ensures standards of care are adhered to, and validates the accountability of each member for mitigating neonatal pain.

The pain committee has primary responsibility for providing information to all health care workers who are responsible for assessing and alleviating neonatal pain using pharmacological and nonpharmacological interventions. Interdisciplinary collaboration becomes key when considering the working knowledge of pharmacological interventions. Pharmacists are educated in pharmacokinetics and pharmacodynamics of pharmaceuticals. Physicians, physician assistants, and advanced practice nurses also have a fundamental understanding of the physiological effect of pharmaceuticals. The contribution from these specialties is imperative for comprehensive management of pain.

Nursing staff and parents have an intimate understanding and knowledge of the behavioral and physiological cues infants present during assessment of pain and are integral to the team. As the primary assessors and deliverers of interventions, the contribution of nurses and families are instrumental in the development of comprehensive, successful pain management plans. Parents and nurses are responsible for delivery of nonpharmacological interventions of pain management and, as committee members, their working understanding of those interventions is paramount in their appropriate use.

Together, each member of the committee should have an understanding of the availability, effect of, and appropriate use of pharmacological and nonpharmacological interventions. Team knowledge of available pharmaceuticals in the organization allows quicker response to pain mitigation from all parties. Knowledge of the effects of the pharmaceutical allows better follow-up assessment from direct caregivers and parents. Appropriate use of nonpharmacological interventions allows synergy of interventions. The pain committee has the responsibility of ensuring each member is accountable for the understanding, availability, and use of available therapies for neonatal pain management.

Cumulative responsibilities of all members of a pain committee are maintaining currency in evidence supporting best-practice standards, education plans for health care staff, process-improvement strategies, and working collaboratively with all members. Inclusion of families allows for individualized care plans and interventions. The committee needs to work collaboratively with families to understand spiritual and cultural beliefs of pain management and to develop appropriate, individualized plans. Implementing the generalized knowledge and processes of the committee as a whole for each family will allow a quality, personalized approach to pain management and improving outcomes (Joint Commission Resources, 2003).

Communication techniques can support the elements of a pain committee, promote the benefits of debriefing, and advance the education of all team members. Good communication techniques also promote family involvement and greater patient or family satisfaction with care delivery and pain management. The elements of good communication techniques require understanding of the three steps of the communication process—the sender, the message, and the receiver. Communication can only occur if the receiver fully understands the message the sender intends to send. The flow of communication is typically what the sender intended to say, what the sender actually said, what the receiver heard, and what the receiver thinks he or she heard. It is imperative to ensure the flow of communication is understood and is working to relay information about the infant's pain, how to manage the pain, and the response to the interventions used.

Health care workers can promote good communication using techniques or processes that support transfer of information comprehensively and completely. AHRQ promotes the use of evidence-based tools, such as call-outs and check-backs, to ensure the message the sender intended is the message the receiver received. Call-outs ensure all team members receive information simultaneously while helping all team members to anticipate the next steps; they also direct responsibility of a specific individual to carry out a specific task (AHRQ, n.d.). Checkbacks close the loop of communication to ensure the information sent is understood. The receiver is required to restate the message sent by the sender for validation, and the sender restates the message to confirm the transfer of correct information. These methods of communication reduce misinterpretation and misunderstanding in communication, promote collaboration, and support best practice. Reducing misunderstanding and misinterpretations of information transfer is fundamental in promote better pain management of neonates, especially when including the parents in the pain management team.

Techniques that can be taught to families so they can communicate pain symptoms of their infant are the call-out and check-back; it is essential to create a safe environment for the families to report their findings. Ensuring language barriers are controlled is a first step in creating that safe environment. Providing tools that are universal will help to encourage family collaboration and communication of assessment findings. Educating the family on the behavioral cues of the infant how to communicate the findings in a nonthreatening and supportive environment helps create a team approach to care and a trusting relationship. Teaching families how to check-back—making sure the communication tools the family is using are fully understood by the health care worker and the information sent back to the family by the health care worker is fully understood—works to promote better pain management. Educating families about neonatal behavioral pain cues is a necessary step in creating a trusting, safe environment that uses universal language and reporting tools that will help families communicate pain symptoms to the health care team.

A multidisciplinary approach to pain management of the neonate is imperative for the best outcome of the infant. Collaboration among all disciplines, an understanding of what each discipline's role is in mitigating pain, and the importance of quality communication processes work together to promote the best outcomes and best pain management of the neonate. The importance of education of health care workers and families, the use of case studies for education and process improvement, the need for pain committees and debriefing cannot be emphasized enough. Following is an example of how good communication techniques during a debriefing session of an interdisciplinary team can promote process improvement for better pain management for future incidences and future infants.

GOOD COMMUNICATION TECHNIQUES

SCENARIO ONE

A 40-week, 36-hour-old infant was born via vaginal delivery with thick meconium and was subsequently admitted to NICU for respiratory distress and suspected right-sided pneumothorax. A 5 French chest tube was place anteriorly at 42 hours of life. The mother and father of the infant were at bedside after chest tube insertion and attempting to console the infant, who was grimacing, tachycardic at 180 bpm, tachypneic at 45 breaths per minute, and crying. Both mother and father insisted the infant was in pain and repeatedly questioned the nurse about pain medication and helping their baby to stop crying. The nurse caring for the infant informed the parents that the infant had received pain medication at the time of chest tube insertion and would calm down soon. The mother was crying and the father was getting very upset. The father insisted the physician present at the bedside and demanded to speak to the nurse in charge. The physician presented at the bedside, ordered a stat dose of intravenous (IV) pain medication, which the nurse subsequently administered. Within 10 minutes, the infant's heart rate was 160 bpm, respirations were 30, facial expression was calm, and the infant was falling asleep as his mother held his hand. The father insisted on a conversation with the charge nurse, physician, and bedside nurse. The director of nursing (DON) for the NICU arranged for a parent meeting within the hour in a conference room within the unit, away from the bedside. The following debrief conversation occurred with the team as they used the debriefing checklist presented earlier.

The DON inquires as to whether the family felt communication between themselves and the health care team was clear.

The DON understands the importance of ensuring and promoting clear, timely communication among all members of the health care team and ensuring protocols are adhered to for ensuring patient safety and comfort.

The physician understands the parents were concerned about the acute pain the child was experiencing. The physician further understands that the nurse communicated that the infant was in pain and the parents were requesting pain medication at the time of the chest tube insertion. The physician does not understand what the parent's role could be in making sure the child stayed pain free.

The nurse understands her role in educating the family in how to assess and report their child's pain and being a stronger advocate in requesting that the physician manage the pain faster. The nurse understands her role in bridging the gap of communication between the interdisciplinary team and being an advocate for the patient and the family.

The pharmacy staff understands the role in ensuring requested medication is delivered in a timely fashion to the NICU for administration during or before painful procedures. The pharmacy staff understands the importance of stat dosing of medications and the need to dispense and deliver medication as quickly as possible.

The family understands their role in advocating for their child, communicating with appropriate language and tone to promote teamwork to ensure their child is pain free. The family understands the need to request education, inclusion, and to acknowledge teamwork when good communication exists.

SCENARIO TWO

A 31-week, 20-day-old infant is 8 days postop from a complicated abdominal surgery for necrotizing enterocolitis with a jejunal stoma and mucus fistula. The infant received a continuous fentanyl drip immediately for 5 days postop and was vigorously weaned off pain medication on day 6. On day 8, the infant is irritable, with a heart rate consistently in the 180s, is tachypneic with respirations at 50 on continuous positive airway pressure, exhibits guarding with abdominal auscultation and diaper changes, and is grimacing with concomitant nasolabial furrowing. The parents are at the bedside requesting the nurse administer pain medication. The nurse informs the family no pain medication is ordered for the infant and that a facilitated tuck and reducing stimuli will be sufficient. The mother insists pain medication be ordered and administered while the father insists the physician assess his child. The nurse alerts the covering physician of the parents' concerns and she presents at the bedside. The father adamantly insists pain medication be ordered and given to his child, while the mother begins to become visibly distraught over her child's signs of pain. The physician is reluctant to order pain medication and attempts to explain the risks of respiratory depression and the use of non-pharmacological interventions to manage pain. The parents become even more upset as the infant's vital signs continue to show tachycardia and tachypnea and the infant begins crying. The parents begin to demand a transfer of the infant to an institution that will listen to their concerns and manage the infant's pain. The bedside nurse alerts the DON of the escalating situation, who immediately calls a family meeting with the covering case manager, physician, family, and nurse. Using the debriefing checklist, the following debriefing conversation occurred with the family and health care team.

The DON inquires as to whether the family feels communication between themselves and the team was clear. The DON understands the importance of ensuring and promoting clear, timely communication among all members of the health care team and ensuring protocols are adhered to for ensuring patient safety and comfort. The parents are adamant because the communication is not clear and their concerns for the child's pain are not being considered.

The physician understands the parents' concern about the acute pain that the child is experiencing. The physician further understands the communication with the nurse that the infant was in pain and the parents were requesting pain medication.

The physician was not clear what the parents' role could be in making sure their child stayed pain free or indicating that the infant was demonstrating acute signs of pain that affected his or her vital signs. The physician was not receptive to the family or nursing staff suggestions to mitigate the infant's pain with pharmacological interventions.

The nurse understands her role in educating the family on how to assess and report their child's pain and to be a stronger advocate to the physician for managing pain. The nurse understands her role in bridging the gap of communication between the interdisciplinary team and being an advocate for the patient and the family.

The workload distribution is not a concern in this scenario.

The bedside nurse requested task assistance from the DON seeking, intervention and mediation between the physician and the family in addressing the emotional distress the parents were experiencing and developing an amicable resolution. The DON immediately understood the seriousness of the situation and the need to find a reasonable and agreeable resolution to promote family satisfaction and end to de-escalate an emotionally charged scenario. The DON understands case management can be an integral part of the health care team in explaining to families the financial impact of transfers to other facilities of medically fragile patients.

The family understands its role in advocating for the child, communicating with appropriate language and tone to promote teamwork and ensure the child's pain is managed. The nurse and DON understand the role of advocate for patient treatment, but also recognize the support the parents need in making decisions and having their concerns addressed. The case manager understands her role in helping to educate the family on the financial impact of decisions made during emotional crisis.

A positive event in this scenario was the bedside nurse's success in de-escalating the situation before parental emotions became unreasonable or unmanageable. The DON recognized the need to bring available resources to the situation and to call

all members together to discuss the concerns and plan of care so as to find a reasonable and agreeable resolution. The team learned that in future situations better communication with families is needed regarding the pain management treatment plan before, during, and after surgery, as well as documenting parental understanding of the risks and benefits of pharmacological pain management.

SCENARIO THREE

A 36-week, 4-day-old infant is demonstrating signs of withdrawal after being born to a mother receiving 100 mg of methadone for the last 15 weeks of pregnancy after a history of heroin use. The infant is tachypneic with respirations of 48, tachycardic at 185 bpm, diaphoretic, is arching his back, has an angry rash across his buttocks, and is extremely irritable and inconsolable. The mother has not visited since day 2 and nursing staff have not been successful in securing a reliable method of communication with the mother or other family members. The nursing staff have provided the infant with clothing, blankets, and a quiet space with limited environmental stimulation. As day 4 progresses, the infant's symptoms continue to escalate with vomiting after feeds. The assigned nurse alerts the covering physician of the worsening symptoms, suggesting pharmacological intervention for reduction of withdrawal symptoms. The first-year pediatric resident responds to the bedside, does a preliminary assessment and determines the infant can be managed with nonpharmacological management and continued assessment. The bedside nurse does not agree and again details the infant's signs and symptoms, including the infant's elevated temperature. The first-year pediatric resident refuses to reconsider, at which time the bedside nurse contacts the resident's superior to assess the infant and review infant history. The third-year resident reviews the maternal history, the infant's history, and agrees to order pharmacological intervention for the infant. Using the debriefing checklist, the following debriefing conversation occurred with the health care team.

The nurse understands her role to advocate for the child's pain and escalates her intervention as necessary to manage pain. The nurse understands her role in ensuring the infant's best interests are managed in the absence of family. The third-year resident understands his role in ensuring optimal care of withdrawal symptoms is managed.

The workload distribution is not a concern in this scenario.

Task assistance was requested by the bedside nurse from the third-year superior resident for intervention and to provide experienced direction to the first-year resident in the best interest of the infant. The physician, as the superior, immediately understood the seriousness of the situation and the need to treat the symptoms of opiate withdrawal to reduce negative physiological impact to the infant. The first-year resident understood the need to respect and defer to the experience of a superior medical team, which contributed to what went well in this situation. What needs to improve is the first-year resident's understanding of when to seek advice while gaining a deeper understanding of opiate withdrawal symptoms of neonates.

REFERENCES

Agency for Healthcare Research and Quality. (n.d.). *TeamSTEPPS*. Retrieved from http://www.ahrq.gov/cpi/about/otherwebsites/teamstepps/teamstepps.html

Boyle, E. M., & McIntosh, N. (2004). Pain and compassion in the neonatal unit—A neonatologist's view. *Neuroendocrinology Letters, 25*(Suppl. 1), 49–55.

Bradshaw, M. J., & Lowenstein, A. J. (2014). *Innovative teaching strategies in nursing and related health professions*. Burlington, MA: Jones & Bartlett.

Friedrichs, J. B., Young, S., Gallagher, D., Keller, C., & Kimura, R. E. (1995). Where does it hurt? An interdisciplinary approach to improving the quality of pain assessment and management in the neonatal intensive care unit. *Nursing Clinics of North America, 30*(1), 143–159.

Herr, K., Coyne, P. J., Key, T., Manworren, R., McCaffery, M., Merkel, S., . . . Wild, L. (2006). Pain assessment in the non-verbal patient: Position statement with clinical practice recommendations. *Pain Management Nursing, 7*(2), 44–52.

Joint Commission Resources. (2003). *Improving the quality of pain management through measurement and action.* Oakbrook Terrace, IL: Author.

Newhouse, R. P., & Spring, B. (2010). Interdisciplinary evidence-based practice: Moving from silos to synergy. *Nursing Outlook, 58*(6), 309–317. doi:10.1016/j.outlook.2010.09.001

Schultz, M., Loughran-Fowlds, A., & Spence, K. (2009). Neonatal pain: A comparison of the beliefs and practices of junior doctors and current best evidence. *Journal of Pediatrics and Child Health, 46*(1-2), 23–28. doi:10.1111/j.1440-1754.2009.01612.x

Walden, M., & Gibbins, S. (2008). *Pain assessment and management guideline for practice* (2nd ed.). Glenview, IL: National Association of Neonatal Nurses.

10

Role of Family in Neonatal Pain Management

The role of the family in neonatal pain management is central and integral to supporting the identification of pain in the neonate, implementating interventions, and promoting the best neurological outcomes of the neonate. The environment of a neonatal critical care unit, which is full of monitors, wires, tubing, beeps, clicks, alarms, interventions, and foreign terminology, is, by itself, more stress than a family anticipates experiencing when discovering a new life is on its way (Heidari, Hasapour, & Foolardi, 2013). Add to the stress of this overwhelming environment the inability to manage even the simplest care for one's newborn—feeding, holding, and positioning—oftentimes a frighteningly small newborn at that. Considering the parental stress in this environment, the loss of control, and the loss of the idea of a perfect delivery and newborn, realizing this fragile new person is experiencing pain can be a trigger point for some families in expressing a lack of coping mechanisms (Obeidat, Bond, & Clark Callister, 2009). Recognizing this loss of control, the stress, and the maternal need to protect, the clinicians should engage the family soon after the admission on how to identify signs of pain, how to deliver nonpharmacological interventions to alleviate or mitigate pain, while working to promote a strong family unit and a satisfactory experience in an otherwise unpleasant situation.

PARENT UNDERSTANDING

Understanding the family's interpretation of pain cues and infant responses to interventions is an important first step in promoting a positive experience for everyone. Families who are educated about the behavioral and physiological cues of neonatal pain will be more inclusive members of the health care team while enjoying a more satisfying experience in the neonatal intensive care unit (NICU). Teaching parents the physiological cues may be the first step in helping the mother and the father understand the equipment and monitors. Helping parents understand the normal parameters of heart rate, respiration, and oxygen saturation for the infant will help them identify when an abnormality exists. Teach the family how to assess what may be a contributing factor to a change in vital signs—opening the portholes and speaking too loudly to the infant may cause a change in oxygenation status—indicate the need for lowered voices, with talking reduced to a minimum. Instruct them that a light, tickling touch on the infant's extremities causes bradycardia and desaturation and that firm, containment touch is supportive for the fragile infant. Ensure that the infant receives nonpharmacological and sucrose support prior to all interventions to prevent physiological instability. When the family gains this level of understanding of thir neonate, their level of empowerment for driving the infant's care increases, providing a greater sense of parenting and satisfaction. The family at the bedside that recognizes the smallest alteration in stability promotes better outcomes for the infant as well.

PARENT EDUCATION

Strategies for helping parents understand and recognize the physiological changes include encouraging frequent visitation through open visiting hours, encouraging parents to participate in daily rounds, encouraging parents to participate in the change-of-shift report, and encouraging skin-to-skin contact, as well as education. Encouraging parents to be present at the bedside as often and for as long as possible helps the parent to know the infant. Infants who go home with their parents are cared for 24/7 by the mother and the father. The family becomes attuned to the cues and behaviors of the infant through this constant bonding contact. The mother becomes attuned to the differences in the infant's cry and what each means. The parents of a NICU infant do not have that proximity to the infant to learn these cues and frequently the infant is so medically fragile he or she is not able to provide the same cues. However, this does not mean the mother and father cannot learn their infant in a different way. Knowing the infant can only occur through regular visits with meaningful time spent at the bedside.

Encouraging that meaningful time at the bedside means providing an environment that supports time spent at the bedside. Liberal visiting hours with limited restrictions on when and how long to visit promote an environment in which the family is welcomed to be present. Allowing parents to visit 24/7 and to spend unrestricted time at the bedside promotes a sense of knowing what is normal and not normal for the child. Transitioning to single-family rooms instead of open-unit concepts can promote the comfort of the family in sitting at the bedside, with less distraction from other patient's monitors, alarms, and general medical activity. Single-family rooms promote privacy and limit environmental distractions.

PARENTS AND ROUNDING

Including the family in daily rounds is another strategy to promote family inclusion in pain management of the neonate. Consistency with time of rounds each day allows the family the opportunity to be present during rounds, even after the mother has been discharged. Participation in daily rounds allows the family to provide valuable input in assessment findings not always recognized by the nurse caring for other patients. Daily rounds allow the family an opportunity to ask questions, gain clarification of behaviors, and provide input for what they believe contributes to or alleviates pain in their infant. Providing this opportunity for inclusion allows a sense of control, which can promote the bonding process and contribute to outcomes that are more positive.

Encouraging parental inclusion at change of shift can go a long way toward promoting better recognition and management of neonatal pain. The family who is spending time at the bedside, learning and recognizing the physiological and behavioral cues of pain, is able to contribute to the shift report thereby promoting care of the infant when they are not present. The family spending time at the bedside can provide more detailed, real-time accounting of any change in physiological stability with an account of what contributed to the change and what resolved it. The family included in bedside shift reporting can be real-time reporters of the 12-hour happenings. Aside from empowering the family in contributing to the daily care plan of the infant, it also promotes a sense of empowerment, again leading to better outcomes and greater satisfaction. The family who is present and contributing will have a better sense of understanding the infant, which eliminates the step of getting to know each other after discharge. This can potentially reduce the number of frantic phone calls back to the unit after. Providing the opportunity for the family to get to know the infant and his or her cues during the hospital stay contributes to better outcomes for all.

Skin-to-skin contact is the best method for the mother and father to learn to promote bonding with the infant. Placing the infant's bare skin on the mother/father's bare skin for periods of no less than 45 minutes, even encouraging this contact for hours at a time is beneficial for the infant in providing physiological stability, reducing glucose and oxygen utilization, and promoting greater breast-milk production for the mother. Focusing the parent's attention on the infant in such intimate proximity allows the parent to learn not only physiological cues but behavioral cues as well. Smell, movement, and sleep cycles during skin-to-skin time contribute to a deeper knowing of the infant by the parent, which either parent can achieve. The benefit of promoting milk production in the mother is an added bonus.

Educating the parents on normal physiological values based on gestational age can help them understand what is normal. Teaching parents the normal parameters of heart rate, respiration, and oxygen saturation as the infant matures helps parents identify the cause when a change occurs. Teaching the parents normal parameters in relation to gestational age increments as the bedside nurse understands them helps the parents better understand where the infant should be. With this added knowledge, parents can be taught to look for environmental events that contribute to change. When parents understand the norms, they are able to recognize what precipitates a change and collaborate to reduce or eliminate it from occurring again. Education is key in all aspects of promoting outcomes and parenting; identifying precipitators of pain and physiological alterations can promote the family bonding as well as good infant outcomes.

Heart rate for the preterm infant ranges from 120 to 170 beats per minute, with the range becoming lower as the gestational age increases (Dieckmann, Brownstein, & Gausche-Hill, 2000). As the infant approaches corrected term or term, a heart rate range of 100 to 120 beats per minute is acceptable (Dieckmann et al., 2000). Respiration for the preterm infant should remain constant from 23 weeks through term or postterm at 40 to 60 breaths per minute. Oxygen saturation by gestational age continues to be a subject of controversy (Chang, 2011). A range from 88% to 98% along a gestational age continuum from 23 weeks gestation to term gestational ages the acceptable target range; however, each individual unit may prefer its own set of vital sign limits as noted in unit policies. Parental education must be based upon each unit's policy and practice language. Parents must learn the stressors that compromise the unit's chosen parameters so they may better advocate for their removal.

Parents need to learn to recognize the stressors that contribute to alterations in the accepted ranges of the infant's physiological stability. Time spent at the bedside can help parents do that. Time spent can help them identify with assurance that every time a particular staff person or activity is encountered, the infant responds consistently in an unstable manner. Recognizing that unstable behavior or alteration in behavior is crucial in preventing it from happening again. Parents need to be encouraged to recognize this and feel empowered to contribute this information to the team. Once we can teach the family to recognize and be confident in the recognition, we can teach them not only how to advocate for but also how to implement nonpharmacological methods of helping the infant survive the stressors.

NONPHARMALOGICAL INTERVENTIONS

Nonpharmacological interventions that we can readily teach families to implement include holding containment, reducing stimuli, and providing nonnutritive sucking. Teaching parents about holding containment to support neurological stability translates to better pain management. When provided with the appropriate education, there is a rare parent who would decline the opportunity to independently deliver interventions aimed at supporting their infant. Teaching parents to provide interventions independently is crucial to preventing escalating physiological instability. Setting limits of what is appropriate for the parent to do and when to notify the bedside clinician is imperative to ensure the safety of the infant. Teaching parents how to identify the limits of physiological stability of their infant to escalate interventions to a pharmacological level promotes a more collaborative approach to pain management and promotes the safety of the infant. Educating the parent to be an advocate in ensuring pharmacological intervention, such as sucrose administration, for all interventions, even heel sticks for glucose screening, promotes autonomy and empowerment of the family.

LEARNING BEHAVIORAL CUES

Teaching parents behavioral cues so they can recognize the pain cues of the infant is as important as understanding the physiological cues. Educating the parents to communicate with the infant and to recognize when the infant is telling them he or she needs help through his or her behaviors contributes to satisfaction and empowerment of the family. Helping parents understand the baby's awake and sleep states, when best to interact with the infant, and how to identify through behavior before physiological alterations occur helps protect the infant from negative outcomes. Parents require education on how to "read" their infant's behaviors, from hand splaying, to gaze aversion, and sneezing, to understand these behaviors are cues that a stressful environment exists and the infant may experience pain as a result. Remembering to teach the parent that the sensation of pain is not only something that causes physical discomfort, but is also an unpleasant sensory or emotional experience is crucial.

When helping parents understand the behavioral cues, the nurse must consider the parent's language, culture, and cognitive maturity and ability. Providing written materials, pictures, or oral instruction with methods of validating understanding helps to ensure the family receives the education in a method that meets individual needs. The nurse being present at the bedside when an infant displays negative behaviors; pointing out those behaviors in real time helps the parent to recognize future demonstrations. These opportunities occur more readily when parents are encouraged to be present, visit frequently, and participate in skin-to-skin care on a regular basis. Promoting the same behaviors and environmental examples when teaching parental recognition of physiological cues will support parental understanding of behavioral cues.

Parent involvement in mitigating pain and their inclusion as part of the care team promotes positive outcomes and improves overall pain management. Teaching parents the norms of physiologic and behavioral guidelines with approaches that meet individual language, cultural, and cognitive needs can support a collaborative, cooperative relationship. The infant benefits when effort is expended at the beginning of the infant's journey through the NICU to incorporate and educate the family as part of the care team. Pain is more quickly recognized, is more quickly remedied, the families are more satisfied, and outcomes are improved for everyone.

REFERENCES

Chang, M. (2011). Optimal oxygen saturation in premature infants. *Korean Journal of Pediatrics, 54*(9), 359–362. doi:10.3345/kjp.2011.54.9.359

Dieckmann, R., Brownstein, D., & Gausche-Hill, M. (2000). *Pediatric education for prehospital professionals*. Sudbury, MA: Jones & Bartlett.

Heidari, H., Hasapour, M., & Foolardi, M. (2013). The experiences of parents with infants in the neonatal intensive care unit. *Iranian Journal of Nursing and Midwifery Research, 18*(3), 208–213.

Obeidat, H. M., Bond, E. A., & Clark Callister, L. (2009). The parental experience of having an infant in the newborn intensive care unit. *Journal of Perinatal Education, 18*(3), 23–29.

Special Populations

Procedural Pain Management

There are many reasons a neonate can experience pain. Pain can be caused by trauma (such as a traumatic delivery), a pathological condition or anomaly, or from an invasive procedure.

Table 11.1 describes some of the common painful procedures experienced by the neonate in the neonatal intensive care unit (NICU).

CIRCUMCISION

Male circumcision, or removal of the foreskin or prepuce from the penis, is a common procedure performed on neonates for religious, cultural, or personal reasons. Although circumcision can be performed at any time in life, it is most completely performed during the neonatal period. There has been a move away from performing it in the hospital before a newborn is discharged; it is more commonly performed during a follow-up pediatric visit to ensure the baby has fully transitioned to extrauterine life and that breastfeeding is well established.

Pain management during circumcision varies, with some procedures still receiving no analgesia at all. The American Academy of Pediatrics (AAP) recommends that pharmacological methods be used, as nonpharmacological methods alone are insufficient at managing pain during this procedure. Adequate analgesia, such as topical 4% lidocaine, dorsal penile nerve block (DPNB), and a subcutaneous ring block are all effective options, although the

TABLE 11.1 Common Invasive Procedures in the NICU
Invasiveness
Mild
Insertion of nasogastric or orogastric tube
Physical examination
Umbilical arterial or venous catheter placement
Nose culture
Tracheal suctioning
Bladder catheterization
Eye culture
Auditory evoked potential
Moderate
Arterial puncture
Venous puncture
Venous catheterization
Heel lance
Tracheal intubation
Intramuscular injection
Central venous catheter removal
Thoracentesis
Surfactant administration

(continued)

TABLE 11.1 Common Invasive Procedures in the NICU (*continued*)
Invasiveness
Suture removal
Tracheal extubation
Ventricular tap (percutaneous)
Severe
Arterial/venous cut down
Arterial catheterization
Circumcision
Lumbar puncture
Eye examination for retinopathy
Bronchoscopy or endoscopy
Suprapubic bladder tap
Central venous catheter placement
Chest tube placement
Greater than three attempts at venous catheterization

NICU, neonatal intensive care unit.

Adapted from Anand et al. (2005).

AAP task force found the subcutaneous ring block to be the most effective. The task force also found that infants who were circumcised without analgesia demonstrated an increased behavioral response to routine immunizations at 4 to 6 months compared to infants with adequate pain management (AAP, 2012).

HEEL LANCE

Blood sampling by heel lancing is the most commonly performed neonatal invasive procedure and is reported to be more painful than venipuncture for infants (Larrsson, Tannfeldt, Lagercrantz, & Olsson, 2000). Pain management is essential for this routine procedure. A combination of sucrose and a pacifier and swaddling or facilitated tucking has been reported to be the most effective intervention when performing a heel lance (Gibbins et al., 2002).

INTUBATION

Endotracheal intubation is a common occurrence in the NICU. Because respiratory function is where most of the infants' symptoms will manifest, it is important to establish and maintain a patent airway. Sometimes infants are intubated for medication delivery (such as surfactant) and then immediately extubated, other times a longer duration of airway management and ventilation is needed. Unless the intubation is a true emergency, pain relief is recommended. From review of the research in 2006, it was found that awake intubation (without the use of mediations) was associated with significantly higher intracranial pressure, higher blood pressure, and a more variable heart rate than premedicated intubation (Byrne & Mackinnon, 2006). The treatment is usually an opioid of choice such as morphine or fentanyl. Midazolam (Versed) or another sedative and atropine may be added to the preintubation protocol. A sedative will relax the patient, making intubation easier and more successful and may potentiate the effects of the opioid. Atropine blocks the vagal response that may be elicited by placement of the laryngoscope and endotracheal tube and also minimizes secretions, which will also allow a more successful placement (DeBoer & Peterson, 2001). Dosages of opioids and sedatives are based on weight (see Chapter 4) and atropine is 0.01 to 0.03 mg/kg/dose intravenously (IV) over 1 minute with onset of action in about 2 minutes (DeBoer & Peterson, 2001).

LUMBAR PUNCTURE

Lumbar puncture is commonly performed to obtain spinal fluid and rule out sepsis and/or meningitis. This is a painful procedure and one during which the neonate must remain still in order to successfully obtain a sample. The patient should be tucked as best as possible (with the area of insertion exposed), should have a pacifier and sucrose at minimum. The infant can be premedicated with morphine or fentanyl before the puncture is attempted. Topical or subcutaneous lidocaine or a lidcoaine combination may also be used to manage the pain during insertion (Anand et al., 2005).

SURGERY

Pain management during surgery is imperative. Proper anesthesia and analgesia are important and drug selection depends on the type of surgery, duration of surgery, and the condition of the neonate, among other factors. Pain management should also be continued after surgery, until the patient is no longer exhibiting pain symptoms according to the standardized scale used by the institution in which care is delivered.

VENOUS AND ARTERIAL PUNCTURE

Babies often receive venipuncture for blood samples or when they need to receive intravenous fluids. Arterial samples may be needed or an arterial line placed if monitoring arterial blood gas or blood pressure. All of these procedures are painful and may require several attempts to be successful. All babies should be swaddled and given sucrose. Application of a topical anesthetic cream, such as lidocaine 2.5% and prilocaine 2.5%, may also be used (Anand et al., 2005). For central venous catheter placement or multiple attempts at venipuncture, opioids, topical anesthetics, and benzodiazepines are also sometimes indicated (Anand et al., 2005).

REFERENCES

American Academy of Pediatrics. (2012). Circumcision policy statement, task force on circumcision. *Pediatrics, 130*(3), e756–e785.

Anand, K. J. S., Johnson, C. C., Oberlander, T. F., Taddio, A., Tutag Lehr, V., & Walco, G. A. (2005). Analgesia and local anesthesia during invasive procedures in the neonate. *Clinical Therapeutics, 27*(6), 844–876.

Byrne, E., & Mackinnon, R. (2006). Should premedication be used for semi-urgent or elective intubation in neonates? *Archives of Disease in Childhood, 91*(1), 79.

DeBoer, S., & Peterson, L. (2001). Sedation for non-emergent neonatal intubation. *Neonatal Network, 20,* 19.

Gibbins, S., Stevens, B. J., Hodnett, E., Pinelli, J., Ohlsson, A., & Darlinton, G. (2002). Efficacy of safety of sucrose for procedural pain relief in preterm and term neonates. *Nursing Research, 51,* 375–382.

Larrsson, B. A., Tannfeldt, G., Lagercrantz, H., & Olsson, G. L. (2000). Alleviation of pain of venipuncture in neonates. *Acta Paediatrica, 87,* 774–779.

12

The Premature Infant

Identifying behavioral and physiological cues of pain in premature infants, as well as managing that pain, presents unique challenges. The *premature infant* is defined as a fetus delivered before completing 37 weeks gestation. The premature infant includes those neonates meeting age of viability for gestational development; in many states that gestational age is 23 weeks. The range of physiological and physical maturity in premature babies is broad and provides significant challenges to the health care provider. Neurodevelopmental maturity by gestational age, physiological maturity of organ systems, and physical maturity of visible structures do not always match the neonate's actual capacity to send messages, which creates difficulty in identifying and treating pain. It also further complicates education of the parent. The best approach for assessing, identifying and managing this population is through education of the clinician and the family (Ballard et al., 1991).

Physiological maturity increases by gestational age, beginning at the age of viability: 23 weeks. The 23-week-gestation infant's cardiovascular capacity has a reduced ability to increase contractility of the cardiac tissue, thus a decreased capacity regulates blood flow (Kenner & Lott, 2003). The compensatory response of cardiac tissue causes tachycardia and compromised cerebral perfusion, leading to alterations in blood pressure and mean arterial pressure. Increasing gestational age allows increasing maturity of cardiac musculature, leading to improving cardiac output and perfusion by term gestation. The compromised cardiac output and ensuing alterations in vital signs are interpreted for what they are—unstable vital signs and physiological status, but oftentimes they are not interpreted as vital signals of pain. Tachycardia or hyperthermia are signs of pain in an otherwise stable term newborn—environmental factors for hyperthermia are ruled out and assessment findings lead to an interpretation of pain. Not so for the premature infant. Time spent ensuring cardiac output, volume integrity, and environmental factors delays recognition of pain.

Beginning at the age of viability at 23 weeks gestation, respiratory status of the premature infant requires full respiratory support, including oxygen supplementation. Whereas the full-term infant can exhibit desaturation symptoms during times of pain, the preterm infant again sends misinterpreted cues that delay intervention (Kenner & Lott, 2003; Kenner & McGrath, 2004). In the presence or absence of oxygen supplementation and mechanical support, desaturations in a preterm infant of 23 to 37 weeks gestation directs the clinician to troubleshoot airway and gas exchange. Assessment of patency of invasive airway support, integrity of artificial airways and tubing, percentage of fractioned oxygen support all lead to delays in identifying pain as the mitigating factor for desaturation. The physiological immaturity of the premature infant inhibits its ability to consistently engage in stable gas, which compromises one's capacity to recognize pain cues using physiological markers.

Physiological immaturity related to gestational age affects the renal and gastrointestinal systems as well as the cardiac and respiratory systems. The renal system and gastrointestinal system are not as reliable or involved in sending signs of pain in a preterm or term infant and typically suffer sequelae of pain stimuli in response to cardiac and respiratory compromise from stimulus (Kenner & Lott, 2003). For the purpose of this discussion, renal and gastrointestinal integrity will not be discussed as physiologically important for pain assessment or management in neonates.

Skeletal and muscular integrity matures with increasing gestational age in terms of mass and neurological maturity. Skeletomuscular immaturity at 23 to 25 weeks gestation limits the neonate's capacity to generate flexion, experience smooth range-of-motion movements, and display physical signs of pain or discomfort. The premature infant from 23 to 25 weeks by gestation is normally flaccid, with hands and legs splayed away from the body's core, limiting the clinician's ability to use posturing as a measure of pain or as exhaustion from pain. With increasing gestational maturity, in about 2-week increments, the neonate becomes increasingly able to voluntarily move to physiological flexion—a sign of skeletomuscular maturity in a term newborn. With increasing gestational age, the assessment of degree of physiological flexion allows the clinician to visually observe the capacity to self-stabilize in response to painful stimuli or the inability to do so (Chang, 2011; Dieckmann, Brownstein, & Gausche-Hill, 2000; Friedrichs, Young, Gallagher, Keller, & Kimura, 1995; Gallo, 2003; Heidari, Nasapour, & Foolardi, 2013; Kenner & Lott, 2003; Kenner & McGrath, 2004; Obeidat, Bond, & Clark Callister, 2009).

Neurodevelopmental immaturity compromises the clinician's ability to identify pain responses in the neonate. The extremely premature infant, born between 23 and 25 weeks gestation, is still in the organizational stage of neurological development, with neuronal and glial cell migration not yet complete, myelination of neuronal sheaths and synaptic connections also incomplete (Chang, 2011; Dieckmann, Brownstein, & Gausche-Hill, 2000; Friedrichs, Young, Gallagher, Keller, & Kimura, 1995; Gallo, 2003; Heidari, Nasapour, & Foolardi, 2013; Kenner & Lott, 2003; Kenner & McGrath, 2004; Obeidat, Bond, & Clark Callister, 2009). This degree of immaturity does not allow the neonate to express signs of pain; in reality, it is the time of premature life that the experiential stimulus from the hostile NICU environment is hardwiring the brain to not respond to pain. Extra caution must be taken to reduce external stimuli, such as light, noise, and touch, as much as possible, as each are perceived by the extremely premature infant as painful, unpleasant stimuli. Care must be taken to recreate the protective environment of the uterus the neonate should still be growing in to prevent deleterious brain development.

The immature neurodevelopmental status of the neonate born at less than 32 weeks gestation provides the most challenges when assessing and learning to identify signs and symptoms of pain. Not only is the neuronal capacity of the brain limited in its ability to process stimuli and elicit a response, the skeletomuscular maturity is limited as well, which contributes to a decreasing capacity to display outward signs of pain. The use of a maturity tool to determine neuromuscular and physical maturity of neonates beginning with age of viability through term will help the clinician to determine characteristics of maturity to recognize signs of pain more successfully.

The New Ballard Score tool allows the clinician to assess and determine a gestational age by appearance and behavior, to be able to more fully understand the signs and behaviors of the infant so as to identify pain. Having a deeper understanding of the neurobehavioral capacity of the infant allows better identification of pain cues of the premature infant. Assessing the infant and determining a gestational score using the tool provides a foundation of what the infant is capable of. The first part of the tool, as noted in Figure 12.1, directs the clinician to determine neuromuscular maturity by assessing posture, square window, aim recoil, popliteal angle, scarf sign, and heel to ear. A score is assigned based on the infant's presentation in each category from –1 to 5. Next, the clinician determines physical maturity by assessing skin, lanugo,

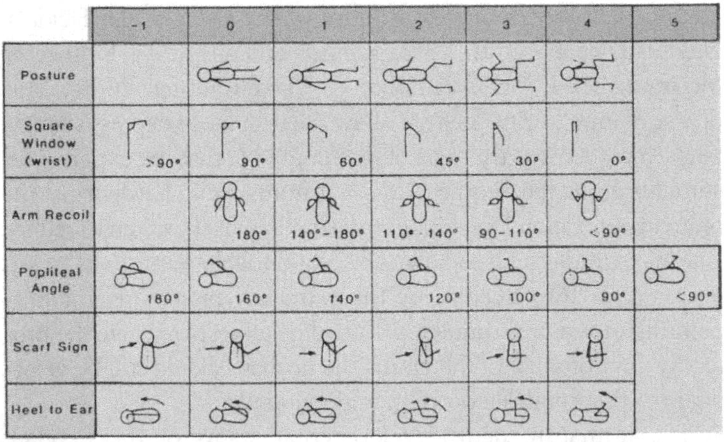

FIGURE 12.1. Neuromusclar maturity.

TABLE 12.1 Physical Maturity as Determined by the New Ballard Score							
	−1	0	1	2	3	4	5
Skin	Sticky, friable, transparent	Gelatinous, red, translucent	Smooth, pink, visible veins	Superficial peeling and/ or rash; few veins	Cracking, pale areas, rare veins	Parchment, deep cracking, no vessels	Leathery, cracked, wrinkled
Lanugo	None	Sparse	Abundant	Thinning	Bald areas	Mostly bald	
Plantar surface	Heel–toe 40–50 mm: −1 < 40 mm: −2	> 50 mm no crease	Faint remarks	Anterior transverse crease only	Creases over anterior 2/3	Crease over entire sole	
Breast	Impercep-tible	Barely perceptible	Flat areola, no bud	Stripped areola, 1–2-mm bud	Raised areola, 3–4-mm bud	Full areola, 5–10-mm bud	
Eye/ Ear	Lids fused loosely: −1 tightly: −2	Lids open, pinna flat, stays folded	Slightly curved pinna; soft slow recoil	Well-curved pinna; soft but ready recoil	Formed and firm; instant recoil	Thick cartilage; ear is stiff	

Maturity rating

Score	Weeks
−10	20
−5	22
0	24
5	26
10	28
15	30
20	32
25	34

(continued)

TABLE 12.1 Physical Maturity as Determined by the New Ballard Score (*continued*)

	-1	0	1	2	3	4	5	
Genitals (male)	Scrotum flat, smooth	Scrotum empty, faint rugae	Testes in upper canal, rare rugae	Testes descending, few rugae	Testes down, good rugae	Testes pendulous, deep rugae		
Genitals (female)	Clitoris prominent, labia flat	Prominent clitoris, small labia minora	Prominent clitoris, enlarging minora	Majora and minora equally prominent	Majora large, minora small	Majora cover clitoris and minora		

Score	Weeks
30	36
35	38
40	40
45	42
50	44

Source: Ballard et al. (1991). Reprinted by permission of Dr. Ballard and Mosby-Year Book, Inc.

plantar surface, breast, eye/ear, and gender genitalia. A descriptive finding in each category is determined, with each earning a score from –1 to 5 as well. The resultant scores for neuromuscular maturity and physical maturity are added together for a total score that correlates with gestational age, as noted on the maturity rating box of Table 12.1. The clinician will now be better able to identify subtle signs and symptoms of pain in premature infants.

Neurobehavioral maturity of an infant progresses in a sequential manner from age of viability to term gestation. The preterm infant has limited capacity to display signs of distress in response to extraneous and negative stimuli. Premature infants have limited reserves for mounting and demonstrating a response. The immature physiological capacity reduces the ability to display or maintain physiological changes in response to painful stimuli. The premature infant is at greater risk of having unrecognized and untreated pain because of an immature capacity to mount and sustain physiological and behavioral signs of pain (Flick & Hebl, 2013).

Premature infants are at the same risk of exposure and experience procedural or postoperative pain as do term infants. The responses are frequently less obvious, less vigorous, and displayed for a shorter length of time, demanding the clinician and family be observant and astute to changes. Encouraging and supporting education of both the clinical caregivers and the family members to know the patient will increase the likelihood that pain is identified and interventions rendered. Encouraging parents to spend time at the bedside, to engage in skin-to-skin care, and to participate in daily rounds increases the parents' ability to "know" the infant. Ensuring clinician education of assessment practices and use of gestational maturity and pain assessment tools promotes earlier recognition of changes. Implementing and enforcing use of a primary care model of care for clinician practice supports the clinical staff in "knowing" the infant's individual cues.

Adoption of an appropriate tool is necessary if the premature infant is to enjoy comprehensive pain management. To date, only two pain tools have modifications for use with premature infants—the Premature Infant Pain Profile (PIPP) and the Neonatal Pain,

Agitation, and Sedation Scale (N-PASS). Although all tools have been used with some reliability with all newborns, the PIPP and N-PASS tools include metrics specific to the premature infant (Flick & Hebl, 2013). Recognizing that the premature infant will experience a degree of pain related to gravity, when term counterparts are weightless in a fluid-filled environment, helps mitigate external sources of tactile sensory stimuli. Recognizing the premature infant's limited capacity to mount a response to constant external stimuli that will result in conditioning of the newborn's fragile and growing neural development is imperative for mitigating pain in the neonate. Recognizing and managing premature infant pain adds a layer of complexity for the clinician in understanding the immaturity of physiological and behavioral responses and then delivering interventions that will be successful.

Interventions for mitigating pain in premature infants must consider the immaturity of the baby's physiological and behavioral states. Position changes using appropriate products, such as snugglies, beanbags, and gel mattresses, can alleviate gravity-related pain responses. Reduction of external stimuli, such as noise and light, can alleviate physiological stimulation and pain. Keep isolettes covered with thick, light-reflective materials to absorb noise and light. Be mindful not to slam porthole doors, not to tap or write on isolettes, to respond to alarms in a timely manner, keep conversations hushed or removed from the bedside. Keep lights dim and cover the baby's eyes during procedures that require brighter lighting. Maintain a neutral thermal environment to reduce metabolic needs to allow for a response to pain. Eliminate noxious smells by removing betadine or alcohol pads and swabs from inside the isolette. Promote the use of colostrum for oral care; provide a pacifier for nonnutritive sucking. Encourage parents to practice skin-to-skin care or teach parents to use facilitated tuck or containment holding when visiting. Administer sucrose as indicated. Administer physician-ordered pharmaceuticals as ordered to control pain. Closely observe vital signs and physical behaviors to recognize signs and symptoms of distress early to contribute to a less painful experience for a premature infant who will grow to have a neurologically stable and healthy brain that has no long-term ill effects because of poorly managed pain during the most crucial and sensitive time of his or her life.

REFERENCES

Ballard, J. L., Khoury, J. C., Wedig, K., Wang, L., Eilers-Walsman, B. L., & Lipp, R. (1991). New Ballard Score, expanded to include extremely premature infants. *Journal of Pediatrics, 119*, 417–423.

Chang, M. (2011). Optimal oxygen saturation in premature infants. *Korean Journal of Pediatrics, 54*(9), 359–362. doi:10.3345/kjp.2011.54.9.359

Dieckmann, R., Brownstein, D., & Gausche-Hill, M. (2000). *Pediatric education for prehospital professionals.* Burlington, MA: Jones & Bartlett.

Flick, R. P., & Hebl, J. R. (2013). Pain management in the postpartum period. *Issues of Clinics in Perinatology, 40*(3), 337–600.

Friedrichs, J. B., Young, S., Gallagher, D., Keller, C., & Kimura, R. E. (1995). Where does it hurt? An interdisciplinary approach to improving the quality of pain assessment and management in the neonatal intensive care unit. *Nursing Clinics of North America, 30*(1), 143–159.

Gallo, A. M. (2003). The fifth vital sign: Implementation of neonatal infant pain scale. *Journal of Obstetric, Gynecologic, & Neonatal Nursing, 32*, 199–206.

Heidari, H., Hasapour, M., & Foolardi, M. (2013). The experiences of parents with infants in the neonatal intensive care unit. *Iranian Journal of Nursing and Midwifery Research, 18*(3), 208–213.

Kenner, C., & Lott, J. W. (2003). *Comprehensive neonatal nursing: A physiological perspective* (3rd ed.). St. Louis, MO: Saunders.

Kenner, C., & McGrath, J. (2004). *Developmental care of newborns and infants: A guide for health professionals.* St. Louis, MO: Mosby.

Obeidat, H. M., Bond, E. A., & Clark Callister, L. (2009). The parental experience of having an infant in the newborn intensive care unit. *Journal of Perinatal Education, 18*(3), 23–29.

Neonatal Abstinence Syndrome

Neonatal drug withdrawal or neonatal abstinence syndrome (NAS) is often a long a painful process that requires time in the neonatal intensive care unit (NICU). Drug withdrawal occurs as the body removes addictive substances from the circulation. It is characterized by central nervous system (CNS) hyperirritability, gastrointestinal dysfunction, respiratory distress, sleep disturbances, and autonomic instability (Finnegan & Kaltenbach, 1992). Untreated NAS can cause significant morbidity and mortality (Finnegan & Kaltenbach, 1992).

NAS may be caused by fetal exposure and dependence in utero or may be iatrogenic (a result of the use of intensive opioid therapy given to the neonate for pain management).

NAS is not new, it has been studied in many forms and is still very common, especially among industrialized nations. Research in 2004 found that 12 out of 1,000 pregnant women used non-prescription drugs and 75 of 1,000 women reported prescription use of analgesics (Wilbourne, Wallerstedt, Dorato, & Curet, 2001). Critically ill patients in the NICU can also experience primary withdrawal from pain medications. Babies may be given consistent morphine or fentanyl because of their diagnosis or perioperatively and then need to be slowly withdrawn from this medication, possibly resulting in NAS symptoms.

Major drugs of abuse include opioids, CNS stimulants, CNS depressants, and hallucinogens, all of which can cause NAS symptoms in the newborn. These symptoms include neurological excitability such as irritability and inability to sleep as well as gastrointestinal effects such as uncoordinated or constant suck, diarrhea, and vomiting (Hudak, Tan, Committee on Drugs, Committee on Fetus and Newborn, & American Academy of Pediatrics, 2012). In a sample of women presenting for drug treatment during pregnancy, more than 89% of neonates experienced NAS that required pharmacological treatment (Woods, 1996).

Iatrogenic withdrawal symptoms have been documented in infants on fentanyl or morphine intravenous drips to maintain continuous analgesia during such therapies as extracorporeal membrane oxygenation (ECMO) and mechanical ventilation (Tobias, 2000).

There are many nonnarcotic drugs that may cause withdrawal symptoms with fetal exposure. Alcohol, barbiturates, caffeine, chlordiazepoxide, clomipramine, diazepam, ethchlorvynol, glutethimide, hydroxyzine, meprobamate, and selective serotonin reuptake inhibitors (SSRIs) are examples (Hudak et al., 2012).

Exposure to drugs during pregnancy has been shown to cause many complications, such as miscarriage, preterm labor, placental abruption, postpartum hemorrhage, malnutrition, anemia, and infections (urinary tract infections or infections often associated with drug abuse such as sexually transmitted diseases). Fetal complications can include intrauterine growth restriction; preterm birth; low birth weight; congenital anomalies; NAS; sudden infant death syndrome; increased incidence of respiratory, ear, and sinus infections; as well as neurologic and behavioral disorders (Behnke, Smith, Committee on Substance Abuse, & Committee on Fetus and Newborn, 2013; Narkowicz, Plotka, Polkowska, Bizuik, & Namiesnick, 2013).

Premature infants may have less severe NAS symptoms compared to term infants. In a study, lower gestational age equated to a lower risk of withdrawal with less severe symptoms when mothers received the same dose of methadone (Liu, Jones, Murray, Cook, & Nanan, 2010). The decrease may be related to a less mature CNS and less fat storage of the drug. This does not mean that the preterm baby will not need treatment. A standardized scale should be used for all babies and treatment given if needed.

Treatment for NAS includes the use of drug therapy to relieve moderate to severe symptoms of withdrawal (Hudak et al.,

2012). Therapy varies with institutional guidelines and provider decision. See Table 13.1 for things to consider when NAS is suspected.

The most common treatments for NAS include opioids (tincture or opium, neonatal morphine, methadone, and paregoric) but barbiturates (phenobarbital), benzodiazepines (diazepam and lorazepam), clonidine, and phenothiazines (chlorpromazine) are often added to the treatment regimen—see Table 13.2 for sample dosages (Hudak et al., 2012). Treatment is usually dependent on careful scoring using a validated NAS scale, such as the Finnegan NAS scale, which is shown in Figure 13.1.

TABLE 13.1 Factors to Consider When NAS Is Suspected
1. What do the results of drug screening show? (Maternal urine, neonatal urine, and neonatal meconium)
2. Does the baby have symptoms?
3. What is the severity of the symptoms according to a tested scale approved by the institution? (Symptoms need to be rechecked frequently according to the guidelines of the scale.)
4. If treatment has begun, is it effective?
5. Can the treatment be weaned? (Again, this is according to institutional policy for weaning. The aim should be to give the least amount of drug that is still effectively assisting with the withdrawal process.)
6. Are social services involved?
7. Is the guardian of this baby involved? (The biological or foster parents should be involved in care as soon as possible. This will both create a smoother transition for discharge and help with the weaning process as they will be able to help with nonpharmacological pain-relief measures.)

NAS, neonatal abstinence syndrome.

TABLE 13.2 Common Treatment Doses for NAS
Morphine
Initial dose: 0.08 mg/kg every 3–4 hr
Titration: Increase by 0.04 mg/kg/dose
Maximum dose: 0.2 mg/kg/dose
Methadone
Initial dose: 0.05–0.1 mg/kg every 6 hr
Tincture of opium
1 mL is added to 24 mL of sterile water to make a concentration equal to that of 0.4 mg of morphine
Initial dose: 0.4 mg by mouth in 6–8 divided doses
Titration: Dose should be increased by 0.04 mg/kg/d or 0.1 mL
Phenobarbital
Initial dose: 20 mg/kg to achieve therapeutic level in one dose
Titration: 10 mg/kg every 12 hr until control or toxicity is noticed
Maintenance dose: 2–6 mg/kg/d for 3–4 day; decrease dose to 3 mg/kg/day
Clonidine
Dose: 0.5–1 mcg/kg every 3 hr with a maximum dose of 1 mcg/kg every 3 hr

NAS, neonatal abstinence syndrome.

Sources: Gardner, Carter, Enzman-Hines, and Hernandez (2011) and Hudak et al. (2012).

SYSTEM	SIGNS AND SYMPTOMS	SCORE	AM 2	4	6	8	10	12	PM 2	4	6	8	10	12	Daily WT.
CENTRAL NERVOUS SYSTEM DISTURBANCES	High Pitched Cry	2													
	Continuous High Pitched Cry	3													
	Sleeps <1 h After Feeding	3													
	Sleeps <2 h After Feeding	2													
	Hyperactive Moro Reflex	2													
	Markedly Hyperactive Moro Reflex	3													
	Mild Tremors Disturbed	2													
	Moderate Severe Tremors Disturbed	3													
	Mild Tremors Undisturbed	1													
	Moderate Severe Tremors Undisturbed	1													
	Increased Muscle Tone	2													
	Excoriation (specific area)	1													
	Myoclonic Jerks	3													
	Generalized Convulsions	1													
METABOLIC/ VASOMOTOR/ RESPIRATORY DISTURBANCES	Sweating	1													
	Fever <101° F(39.3° C)	1													
	Fever > 101°F(39.3° C)	2													
	Frequent yawning (> 3–4 times/interval)	1													
	Mottling	1													
	Nasal stuffiness	1													
	Sneezing (> 3–4 times/interval)	1													
	Nasal flaring	2													
	Respiratory rate > 60/min	1													
	Respiratory rate > 60/min with retractions	2													
GASTROINTESTINAL DISTURBANCES	Excessive sucking	1													
	Poor feeding	2													
	Regurgitation	2													
	Projectile vomiting	3													
	Loose stools	2													
	Watery stools	3													
SUMMARY	TOTAL SCORE														
	SCORERS INITIALS														
	STATUS OF THERAPY														

FIGURE 13.1. Finnegan's NAS scale.

NAS, neonatal abstinence syndrome.
Source: Finnegan (1988). Copyright © Elsevier.

REFERENCES

Behnke, M., Smith, V. C., Committee on Substance Abuse, & Committee on Fetus and Newborn. (2013). Prenatal substance abuse: Short and long term effects on the exposed fetus. *Pediatrics, 131*(3), 1009–1024.

Finnegan, L. P. (1988). Neonatal abstinence syndrome: Assessment and pharmacotherapy. In F. F. Rubehali & N.Grady (Eds.), *Neonatal therapy: An update* (pp. 122–148). New York, NY: Elsevier.

Finnegan, L. P. (1990). Neonatal abstinence syndrome: Assessment and pharmacotherapy. In N. Nelson (Ed.), *Current therapy in neonatal–perinatal medicine* (2nd ed., p. 317). Ontario, Canada: B. C. Decker.

Finnegan, L. P., & Kaltenbach, K. (1992). Neonatal abstinence syndrome. In R. A. Hoekelman, S. B. Friedman, N. M. Nelson, & H. M. Seidel (Eds.), *Primary pediatric care* (2nd ed., pp. 1367–1378). St. Louis, MO: Mosby.

Gardner, S. L., Carter, B. S., Enzman-Hines, M., & Hernandez, J. A. (2011). *Merenstein & Gardner's handbook of neonatal intensive care* (7th ed.). St. Louis, MO: Mosby.

Hudak, M. L., Tan, R. C., Committee on Drugs, Committee on Fetus and Newborn, & American Academy of Pediatrics. (2012). Neonatal drug withdrawl. *Pediatrics, 129*(2), e540–e560.

Liu, A. J., Jones, M. P., Murray, H., Cook, C. M., & Nanan, R. (2010). Perinatal risk factors for the neonatal abstinence syndrome in infants born to women on methadone maintenance therapy. *Australian and New Zealand Journal of Obstetrics and Gynaecology, 50*(3), 253–258.

Narkowicz, S., Plotka, J., Polkowska, Z., Bizuik, M., & Namiesnick, J. (2013). Prenatal exposure to substance abuse: A worldwide problem. *Environmental International, 54*, 141–163.

Tobias, J. D. (2000). Tolerance, withdrawal and physical dependence after long-term sedation and analgesia of children in the pediatric intensive care unit. *Critical Care Medicine, 28*, 6.

Wilbourne, P., Wallerstedt, C., Dorato, V., & Curet, L. B. (2001). Clinical management of methadone dependence during pregnancy. *Journal of Perinatal & Neonatal Nursing, 14*(4), 26–45.

Woods, J. R. (1996). Adverse consequences of prenatal illicit drug exposure. *Current Opinion in Obstetrics and Gynecology, 8*(40), 3–11.

End-of-Life Pain Management and Palliative Care

Although outcomes of survival, overall, in neonatal intensive care units (NICUs) are very favorable, death is also a real part of the NICU experience. The lower the birth weight and earlier the gestation age, the higher the mortality rate. Also, some babies are born with disorders incompatible with life and will not make it through infancy. More common complex or congenital anomalies incompatible with life include trisomy 13, 15, and 18; thanatophoric dwarfism; some errors of inborn metabolism; Potter's syndrome and renal agenesis; severe lung hypoplasia; anencephaly; holoprosencephaly; and some cardiac anomalies (Catlin & Carter, 2002). Kain, Gardner, and Yates (2009) recognize the difficulty in developing and sustaining programs or policies that affect the care of neonates with life-threatening or incompatible life diagnoses and suggest a greater emphasis and more support for doing so. Understanding and managing end-of-life pain and providing palliative interventions are a necessary approach in the NICU.

Palliative care is a necessity for those infants who will not survive premature birth or congenital defects. Providing comfort care for both the infant and his or her family allows the family and the health care team time to emotionally prepare for the baby's death. Although the majority of the research available is about adult end-of-life patients, available data suggest that high-quality end-of-life care for children includes interventions for the relief of pain and other symptoms, usually through pharmacological measures (Institute of Medicine, 2003). Adequate pain relief should be a major goal of end-of-life care. In a retrospective study, researchers found evidence to suggest that palliative drug administration may be driven by the severity of illness; the sicker the patient, the more likely he or she will be treated (Zimmerman et al., 2015). Ensuring policies and protocols are in place for this special population is critically important in managing pain.

Pain management and comfort care should be a major focus for newborns at the end of life, as it is in adults. Health care professionals have a moral and ethical responsibility to ensure adequate pain management during the death of a neonate (Catlin & Carter, 2002). Although the processes and unit-specific management of the environment in which families are provided a peaceful, private place to spend final moments with a terminal infant are beyond the scope of this text, understanding the attention to these factors is important to ensure a good death occurs, so that families can begin a healthy grieving process.

The physiological aspects of pain in neonates with terminal diagnoses are, at best, difficult to determine so the health care team and family are able to provide interventions. Oxygen-saturation monitoring and signs of oxygen starvation can be mis-interpreted; therefore, supplemental oxygen may be delivered in an attempt to provide perceived comfort, whereas delaying or prolonging death may be the result (Caitlin & Carter, 2002). Even with deeper understanding and richer evidence supporting the need for managing neonatal pain to promote neurodevelopmental outcomes, research shows limiting support of neurological management of pain during death (Moura et al., 2011). Research shows a majority of infants reach the end of life receiving ventilator support, antibiotic therapy, and inotropic support but no pain or sedative support (Moura et al., 2011). The National Association of Neonatal Nurses (NANN; 2015) directs neonatal care providers to offer palliative care beginning with the first recognition of life-limiting conditions, to ensure that both the family and infant experience a peaceful, painless, and supportive expiration.

Detailing the elements of the NANN Palliative and End-of-Life Care for Newborns and Infants Position Statement #3063

(2015), palliative care should begin at the same time as curative care when life-limiting conditions are recognized. The goal of palliative care is to incorporate family and health care team voices into a collaborative, appropriate care plan for the infant. The plan should ensure suffering of the neonate is minimal while promoting a shift to comfort care when all benefits of continuing aggressive life-saving interventions are futile and comfort care outweighs the benefit of some interventions. As in adult end-of-life care decisions, ensuring that the peaceful, dignified death of the neonate is preserved should be the focus of palliative care (NANN, 2015). Although this chapter provides more guidance and directives for supporting the family and the importance of implementing standards of care to address palliative care as a process, as opposed to specifically managing neonatal pain, palliative care as a topic in pain management is no less important to address. Neonatal pain is defined as an unpleasant sensory experience and death and dying is certainly an unpleasant sensory experience for both the infant and the family.

NANN position statement #3063 provides guidelines for a model of care addressing end-of-life care of neonates. The first recommendation is to offer palliative care immediately when life-limiting conditions are recognized; whether this be in the delivery room, many days into the NICU stay, or when the infant has been discharged home. Parents who have knowledge of a life-limiting diagnosis prior to delivery should receive palliative care counseling prior to delivery. For families choosing to continue the pregnancy, NANN (2015) suggests family counseling to determine place of birth, who will deliver the infant, who will be present at time of delivery, resuscitation directives are in place, comfort measures are chosen, and spiritual guidance is available.

NANN position statement #3063 (2015) suggests family counseling and family meetings are a critical element of providing comprehensive palliative care for neonates and the parents. Inclusion of the family in all decision-making and explaining conditions, treatment, and options, in easily understood terms, helps the family to make informed decisions and increases understanding of the seriousness of diagnoses. Identifying an advocate for the family prior to delivery or at the time of diagnosis helps the family to provide care and support during the illness time frame and decision-making process. The advocate and health care team must ensure the parents understand the severity, the plan, and the differences between palliative care and end-of-life treatment options if and when an infant must be transferred to a tertiary care center (NANN, 2015). Full disclosure and understanding from the sending institution when transport is necessary helps support grief work for the parents and reduces anger with the receiving institution if different messages are shared with families. Providing written explanations in brochure format and preferably in the family's dominant language helps reinforce verbal counseling.

According to NANN (2015), a palliative care team should include specific members and be able to implement either a palliative care plan or an end-of-life plan of care that is consistent and comprehensive. The palliative care team should include team members whose primary focus is to provide emotional and spiritual support, social workers, chaplains or clergy, a family support specialist for siblings, a parent who has had a child in the NICU, and a lactation consultant. The specialists, social workers, and clergy or chaplains help the family in making decisions, understanding the impact of decisions, and provide ongoing support throughout the process to facilitate understanding and acceptance. The lactation consultant helps the mother donate breast milk if the mother has chosen to begin pumping milk and provide support and guidance in cessation of breast milk production when an infant expires.

The palliative care plan, according to NANN (2015), should include not only curative orders of the neonatal medical management, but also palliative care orders that address discomfort, pain, and gasping or seizure activity. Comfort measures such as skin-to-skin care should be encouraged and supported, for both the mother and the father. Continuing assessment of pain using a validated pain management tool such as the Premature Infant

Pain Profile (PIPP) and providing interventions in the least invasive manner in accordance with results of assessment are a must in managing discomfort and pain. Remembering that palliative care is a supportive approach to managing comfort in life-threatening situations, and is provided concurrently with curative interventions, helps the health care team and family understand that even though life-limiting and life-threatening conditions exist, all hope is not extinguished.

End-of-life plans of care do not include curative interventions and the plans have different goals than those of palliative care plans. According to NANN (2015), the end-of-life plan of care should be set in as private a location as possible, while encouraging and providing space for any family members the parents choose to include. Alarms, pagers, and phones must be turned off within the care area or setting, and lights should be dimmed for family comfort. Harsh clinical lighting, alarms ringing, and phones and pagers buzzing are painful and disruptive signals of life outside the immediate tragedy the family is experiencing. All painful assessments such as heel stick for lab values or blood gases are discontinued and no longer necessary. Frequent assessment of, treatment of, and documentation of pain in the neonate with the unit-chosen pain scale continues without exception when managing an infant in end-of-life scenarios. Parents can be encouraged to provide drops of water or breast milk to the infant for lip lubrication as a comfort measure for not only the infant but for them as well.

End-of-life plans of care should include time and supplies for memory-making activities (NANN, 2015). Bathing and dressing the infant by the family in a private setting with health care team support should be offered. Supporting families in determining who will be present while creating memory boxes, which include handprints and/or footprints, photographs, and locks of hair as well as spiritual ceremonies, is a necessary part of end-of-life care. Families should be supported throughout this process and no family should leave a NICU after an infant expires unescorted. In instances when family cannot be or chooses not to be present for end-of-life care and activities, a staff nurse should hold the infant, bathe and dress him or her, and collect elements of a memory box for the family.

Infants at the end of life should have a health care team member present who provides the family with explanations of what to expect. Explanation of potential gasping, continuing to breathe for minutes to days after withdrawing life support is necessary for parents so that they may have reasonable expectations and understanding of the stages of and natural occurrence of death. Vasopressors and neuromuscular blocking agents should be weaned and discontinued for infants at the end of life, as well as gentle removal of respirator support (NANN, 2015). Nutritional support should also be removed, as artificial nutrition can extend life and prevent the natural dying process. Families must understand and be prepared for death that can take upwards of 3 weeks in some instances when nutritional support is withdrawn.

NANN (2015) suggests palliative and end-of-life care should continue until the infant dies and care should transition to bereavement care at that time. Bereavement care suggestions include providing the infant with a teddy bear so as not to leave with empty arms, following up with phone calls days and weeks after the infant's death, sending cards, contacting the family on the first anniversary of death, offering brochures for support groups, storing memory boxes for up to 1 year for families who decline them at discharge, and/or having memorial events. NANN (2015) also suggests providing debriefing and support services for health care team members for grief support. Throughout all suggested activities and interventions, the key to providing the best support to not only the family but the health care team as well, is communication.

Implementing the steps of the NANN position statement requires deep support and understanding of communication practices and approaches. Ensuring face-to-face discussions with families in quiet, private settings while allowing any persons the family chooses to be present generates an environment of support. Speaking to the families in simple and direct terms about the infant's prognosis helps eliminate any misunderstandings. Telling families in a gentle yet direct manner that death is imminent and care will be rendered although without a cure is necessary (Mancini, Uthaya, Beardsley, Wood, & Modi, 2014.).

Ensure translator services are available to reduce fear and confusion, if necessary, so parents may be well informed and notified. The decision when to withdraw life support should be made with the parents, and the parents should have the option to be present, have other family members present, and to hold the infant before, during, and after death. Parents should be well informed about what to expect as the infant is dying, such as color changes and gasping breaths. Parents should be encouraged to have an opportunity to have spiritual representation and ritual ceremonies performed before, during, and after death (Mancini et al., 2014). Family involvement is paramount in promoting a peaceful passing of any neonate.

Promoting pain management and comfort during the end of an infant's life is controversial when considering the implications of hastening death with the use of narcotic pain medication (Mancini et al., 2014). A deeper understanding of the necessity of pain management is imperative to ensure infants can die with dignity and peace. Some considerations to move care in that direction include use of valid pain scales to measure pain and selection of pain medication. Medication should be administered in the least invasive manner, with buccal or subcutaneous administration preferred (Mancini et al., 2014). Nonnarcotic medications should be administered in conjunction to narcotic medications and nonpharmacological interventions should be incorporated. Swaddling, reducing noise and light stimulation, non-nutritive sucking, massage, and soft music can all support a peaceful death for the infant.

The most common drugs used for end-of-life neonatal care are morphine and fentanyl, which may be used at a higher dose or for a longer term when addressing end-of-life pain management (Moura et al., 2011). This is not because of a lack of consideration for adverse effects, rather the main goal of palliative care is to keep the patient comfortable until death. Meeting the recommendations of NANN position statement #3063 and recognizing the ethical and moral considerations frequently reserved for the adult population should be the same priority with this population as it is for those infants without life-limiting conditions.

Ensuring appropriate developmental and environmental considerations for sound, light, and touch should be a priority, as should using appropriate pain tools to measure pain. Addressing results of chosen pain tools can prevent or reduce negative effects of pain even at the end of life (Moura et al., 2011). Limiting uncomfortable procedures and interventions, such as suctioning, needlesticks, and reintubation, can prevent suffering from unnecessary pain caused by futile activities. End-of-life and palliative care are necessary and ethical considerations when managing all neonates and their families in all aspects of pain management across the continuum of life.

Other medications for consideration when meeting pain management needs of the dying infant can include phenobarbital, midazolam, and diazepam. Each provides relief for any seizure activity that may occur during the dying process, while contributing to the overall pain management of the infant. Dosing is dependent on size and weight of the infant, and delivery is via intravenous route. Ideally, these medications are in addition to morphine and/or fentanyl, and nonpharmacological interventions. Palliative and end-of-life pain management can be addressed with thoughtful use of pharmacological and nonpharmacological interventions, with a short list of pharmaceutical choices. Health care teams must have a deeper understanding of the emotional and psychological elements of neonatal death and dying when addressing pain management needs in neonates. Family awareness with frank, open communication promotes a supportive environment for the infant where pain management can be the focus. Incorporating the family into the decision-making process from the first step of the palliative and end-of-life processes can ensure that the primary focus for the infant is to facilitate a peaceful, dignified, pain-free passing.

REFERENCES

Catlin, A., & Carter, B. (2002). Creation of a neonatal end-of-life palliative care protocol. *Journal of Perinatology, 22*(3), 184–195. Retrieved from http://www.nature.com/jp/journal/v22/n3/full/7210687a.html

Institute of Medicine. (2003). *When children die: Improving palliative and end-of-life care for children*. Washington, DC: National Academies Press.

Kain, V., Gardner, G., & Yates, P. (2009). Neonatal palliative care attitude scale: Development of an instrument to measure the barriers to and facilitators of palliative care in neonatal nursing. *Pediatrics, 123*(2), 207–213. Doi: 10.1542/peds.2008–2774.

Mancini, A., Uthaya, S., Beardsley, C., Wood, D., & Modi, N. (2014). *Practical guidance for the management of palliative care on neonatal units*. Chelsea and Westminster Hospital NHS Foundation Trust.

Moura, H., Costa, V., Rodrigues, M., Almeida, F., Maia, T., & Guimaraes, H. (2011). End of life in the neonatal intensive care unit. *Clinics, 66*(9), 1569–1572. doi:10.1590/S1807-593220110009000011

National Association of Neonatal Nurses. (2015). *Palliative and end-of-life care for newborns and infants position statement #3063*. Retrieved from http://www.nann.org/uploads/files/PalliativeCare6_FINAL.pdf

Zimmerman, K. O., Hornik, C. P., Ku, L., Watt, K., Loughon, M. M., Bidegain, M., . . . Smith, P. B. (2015). Sedatives and analgesics given to infants in neonatal intensive care units at the end of life. *Journal of Pediatrics, 167*(2), 299–304. doi:10.1016/j.jpeds.2015.04.059

Appendix A

Pain Scales

CRIES Pain Scale	DATE/TIME					
Crying—Characteristic cry of pain is high pitched 0—No cry or cry that is not high-pitched 1—Cry high pitched but baby is easily consolable 2—Cry high pitched but baby is inconsolable						
Requires O$_2$ for SaO$_2$ < 95%—Babies experiencing pain manifest decreased oxygenation. Consider other causes of hypoxemia, (e.g., oversedation, atelectasis, pneumothorax) 0—No oxygen required 1— < 30% oxygen required 2— > 30% oxygen required						
Increased vital signs (BP and HR)—Take BP last as this may awaken child making other assessments difficult 0—Both HR and BP unchanged or less than baseline 1—HR or BP increased but increases < 20% of baseline 2—HR or BP is increased > 20% over baseline						

Expression—The facial expression most often associated with pain is a grimace. A grimace may be characterized by brow lowering, eyes squeezed shut, deepening naso-labial furrow, or open lips and mouth 0—No grimace present 1—Grimace alone is present 2—Grimace and non-cry vocalization grunt is present		
Sleepless—Scored based upon the infant's state during the hour preceding the recorded score 0—Child has been continuously asleep 1—Child has awoken at frequent intervals 2—Child has been awake constantly		
TOTAL SCORE		

BP, blood pressure; HR, heart rate; SaO$_2$, oxygen saturation.

From Krechel and Bildner (1995). Reprinted with permission.

Neonatal Infant Pain Scale (NIPS)			
NIPS	0 point	1 point	2 points
Facial expression	Relaxed	Contracted	-
Cry	Absent	Mumbling	Vigorous
Breathing	Relaxed	Different than basal	-
Arms	Relaxed	Flexed/stretched	-
Legs	Relaxed	Flexed/stretched	-
Alertness	Sleeping/calm	Uncomfortable	-

Note: Maximal score of seven points, considering pain ≥ 4.

From Lawrence et al. (1993). Copyright 1993 by Springer Publishing Company. Reprinted with permission.

N-PASS Pain Scale

N-PASS: Neonatal Pain, Agitation, & Sedation Scale

Assessment Criteria	Sedation		Sedation/Pain	Pain/Agitation	
	−2	−1	0/0	1	2
Crying Irritability	No cry with painful stimuli	Moans or cries minimally with painful stimuli	No sedation/ No pain signs	Irritable or crying at intervals Consolable	High-pitched or silent-continuous cry Inconsolable
Behavior State	No arousal to any stimuli No spontaneous movement	Arouses minimally to stimuli Little spontaneous movement	No sedation/ No pain signs	Restless, squirming Awakens frequently	Arching, kicking Constantly awake or Arouses minimally/no movement (not sedated)

(continued)

N-PASS Pain Scale (continued)

N-PASS: Neonatal Pain, Agitation, & Sedation Scale

Assessment Criteria	Sedation		Sedation/Pain	Pain/Agitation	
	-2	-1	0/0	1	2
Facial Expression	Mouth is lax No expression	Minimal expression with stimuli	No sedation/ No pain signs	Any pain expression intermittent	Any pain expression continual
Extremities Tone	No grasp reflex Flaccid tone	Weak grasp reflex ↓ muscle tone	No sedation/ No pain signs	Intermittent clenched toes, fists or finger splay Body is not tense	Continual clenched toes, fists, or finger splay Body is tense
Vital signs HR, RR, BP, SaO_2	No variability with stimuli Hypoventilation or apnea	< 10% variability from baseline with stimuli	No sedation/ No pain signs	↑ 10%–20% from baseline SaO_2 76%–85% with stimulation—quick ↑	↑ > 20% from baseline SaO_2 ≤ 75% with stimulation—slow ↑ Out of sync/fighting vent

Premature Pain Assessment → + 1 if < 30 weeks gestation/corrected age

BP, blood pressure; HR, heart rate; RR, respiratory rate; SaO_2, oxygen saturation.

ASSESSMENT OF SEDATION

- Sedation is scored in addition to pain for each behavioral and physiological criteria to assess the infant's response to stimuli

- Sedation does not need to be assessed/scored with every pain assessment/score

- Sedation is scored from $0 \rightarrow -2$ for each behavioral and physiological criteria, then summed and noted as a negative score $(0 \rightarrow -10)$

  - A score of 0 is given if the infant has no signs of sedation, does not under-react

- Desired levels of sedation vary according to the situation

  - "Deep sedation" $\rightarrow$ goal score of -10 to -5

  - "Light sedation" $\rightarrow$ goal score of -5 to -2

  - Deep sedation is not recommended unless an infant is receiving ventilatory support, related to the high potential for hypoventilation and apnea

ASSESSMENT OF PAIN/AGITATION

- Pain assessment is the fifth vital sign – assessment for pain should be included in every vital sign assessment

- Pain is scored from $0 \rightarrow +2$ for each behavioral and physiological criteria, then summed

  - Points are added to the premature infant's pain score based on the gestational age to compensate for the limited ability to behaviorally communicate pain

  - Total pain score is documented as a positive number $(0 \rightarrow +11)$

- Treatment/interventions are suggested for scores > 3

  - Interventions for known pain/painful stimuli are indicated before the score reaches 3

- The goal of pain treatment/intervention is a score ≤ 3

- More frequent pain assessment indications

  - Indwelling tubes or lines which may cause pain, especially with movement (e.g. chest tubes) $\rightarrow$ at least every 2–4 hours

■ A negative score without the administration of opioids/sedatives may indicate:

  ■ The premature infant's response to prolonged or persistent pain/stress

  ■ Neurologic depression, sepsis, or other pathology

■ Receiving analgesics and/or sedatives → at least every 2–4 hours

  ■ 30-60 minutes after an analgesic is given for pain behaviors to assess response to medication

  ■ Post-operative → at least every 2 hours for 24–48 hours, then every 4 hours until off medications

Paralysis/Neuromuscular Blockade

■ It is impossible to behaviorally evaluate a paralyzed infant for pain

■ Increases in heart rate and blood pressure at rest or with stimulation may be the only indicator of a need for more analgesia

■ Analgesics should be administered continuously by drip or around-the-clock dosing

  ■ Higher, more frequent doses may be required if the infant is post-op, has a chest tube, or other pathology (such as NEC) that would normally cause pain

  ■ Opioid doses should be increased by 10% every 3-5 days as tolerance will occur without symptoms of inadequate analgesia

SCORING CRITERIA

CRYING/IRRITABILITY

−2 → No response to painful stimuli
- No cry with needle sticks
- No reaction to ETT or nares suctioning
- No response to care giving

−1 → Moans, sighs, or cries (audible or silent) minimally to painful stimuli, e.g. needle sticks, ETT or nares suctioning, care giving

0 → No sedation signs or no pain/agitation signs

+1 → Infant is irritable/crying at intervals—but can be consoled
- If intubated—intermittent silent cry

+2 → Any of the following
- Cry is high-pitched
- Infant cries inconsolably
- If intubated—silent continuous cry

EXTREMITIES/TONE

−2 → Any of the following
- No palmar or plantar grasp can be elicited
- Flaccid tone

−1 → Any of the following
- Weak palmar or plantar grasp can be elicited
- Decreased tone

0 → No sedation signs or No pain/agitation signs

+1 → Intermittent (< 30 seconds duration) observation of toes and/or hands as clenched, or fingers splayed
- Body is *not* tense

+2 → Any of the following
- Frequent (≥ 30 seconds duration) observation of toes and/or hands as clenched, or fingers splayed
- Body is tense/stiff

BEHAVIOR/STATE

−2 → Does not arouse or react to any stimuli

- Eyes continually shut or open
- No spontaneous movement

−1 → Little spontaneous movement, arouses briefly and/or minimally to any stimuli

- Opens eyes briefly
- Reacts to suctioning
- Withdraws to pain

0 → No sedation signs or No pain/agitation signs

+1 → Any of the following

- Restless, squirming
- Awakens frequently/easily with minimal or no stimuli

+2 → Any of the following

- Kicking
- Arching

VITAL SIGNS: HR, BP, RR, & O_2 SATURATIONS

−2 → Any of the following

- No variability in vital signs with stimuli
- Hypoventilation
- Apnea
- Ventilated infant—no spontaneous respiratory effort

−1 → Vital signs show little variability with stimuli—less than 10% from baseline

0 → No sedation signs or No pain/agitation signs

+1 → Any of the following

- HR, RR, and/or BP are 10–20% above baseline
- With care/stimuli infant desaturates minimally to moderately (SaO_2 76–85%) and recovers quickly (within 2 minutes)

+2 → Any of the following

- HR, RR, and/or BP are > 20% above baseline

- Constantly awake
- No movement or minimal arousal with stimulation (not sedated, inappropriate for gestational age or clinical situation)

FACIAL EXPRESSION

−2 → Any of the following

- Mouth is lax
- Drooling
- No facial expression at rest or with stimuli

−1 → Minimal facial expression with stimuli

0 → No sedation signs or No pain/agitation signs

+1 → Any pain face expression observed intermittently

+2 → Any pain face expression is continual

- With care/stimuli infant desaturates severely ($SaO_2 < 75\%$) and recovers slowly (> 2 minutes)
- Out of sync/fighting ventilator

© Loyola University Health System, Loyola University Chicago (2009). Pat Hummel, MA, APN, NNP, PNP. Reprinted with permission.

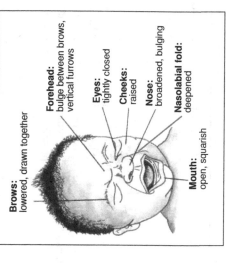

Brows:
lowered, drawn together

Forehead:
bulge between brows, vertical furrows

Eyes:
tightly closed

Cheeks:
raised

Nose:
broadened, bulging

Nasolabial fold:
deepened

Mouth:
open, squarish

Facial expression of physical distress and pain in the infant.

Reproduced with permission from Wong DL, Hess CS: Wong and Whaley's Clinical Manual of Pediatric Nursing, Ed. 5, 2000, Mosby, St. Louis

Premature Infant Pain Scale

Indicators	0	1	2	3
GA in weeks	≥ 36 weeks	32 to 35 weeks and 6 days	28 to 31 weeks and 6 days	< 28 weeks
Observe the NB for 15sec				
Alertness	Active Awake Opened eyes Facial movements present	Quiet Awake Opened eyes No facial movements	Active Sleep Closed eyes Facial movements present	Quiet Sleeping Closed eyes No facial movements
Record HR and SpO₂				
Maximal HR	↑ 0 to 4 bpm	↑ 5 to 14 bpm	↑ 15 to 24 bpm	↑ ≥ 25 bpm
Minimal Saturation	↓ 0 to 2.4%	↓ 2.5 to 4.9%	↓ 5 to 7.4%	↓ ≥7.5%
Observe NB for 30 sec				
Frowned forehead	Absent	Minimal	Moderate	Maximal

	Absent	Minimal	Moderate	Maximal
Eyes squeezed				
Nasolabial furrow	Absent	Minimal	Moderate	Maximal

Absent is defined as 0 to 9% of the observation time; minimal, 10% to 39% of the time; moderate, 40% to 69% of the time; and maximal as 70% or more of the observation time. In this scale, scores vary from zero to 21 points. Scores equal or lower than 6 indicate absence of pain or minimal pain; scores above 12 indicate the presence of moderate to severe pain.

BPM, beats per minute; GA, gestational age; HR, heart rate; NB, newborn.

From Stevens, Johnston, Petryshen, and Taddio (1996). Reprinted with permission.

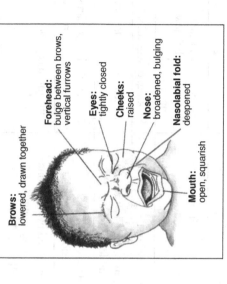

Brows: lowered, drawn together
Forehead: bulge between brows, vertical furrows
Eyes: tightly closed
Cheeks: raised
Nose: broadened, bulging
Nasolabial fold: deepened
Mouth: open, squarish

Facial expression of physical distress and pain in the infant.

Reproduced with permission from Wong DL, Hess CS: Wong and Whaley's Clinical Manual of Pediatric Nursing. Ed. 5, 2000, Mosby, St. Louis

FLACC Pain Scale

Categories	Scoring		
	0	1	2
Face	No particular expression or smile; disinterested	Occasional grimace or frown, withdrawn	Frequent to constant frown, clenched jaw, quivering chin
Legs	Normal position or relaxed	Uneasy, restless, tense	Kicking, or legs drawn up
Activity	Lying quietly, normal position, moves easily	Squirming, shifting back and forth, tense	Arched, rigid, or jerking
Cry	No cry (awake or asleep)	Moans or whimpers; occasional complaint	Crying steadily, screams or sobs, frequent complaints
Consolability	Content, relaxed	Reassured by occasional touching, hugging, or talked to. Distractable	Difficult to console or comfort

Each of the five categories (F) Face; (L) Legs; (A) Activity; (C) Cry; (C) Consolability is scored from 0–2, which results in a total score between 0 and 10.

The FLACC scale was developed by Sandra Merkel, MS, RN; Terri Voepel-Lewis, MS, RN; and Shobha Malviya, MD, at C. S. Mott Children's Hospital, University of Michigan Health System, Ann Arbor, MI. Used with permission. Copyright the Regents of the University of Michigan.

Appendix **B**

Conversion Tables

Weight Conversion Table			
Weight			
Grams	**Ounces**	**Grams**	**Ounces**
10 g	¼ oz	375 g	13 oz
15 g	½ oz	400 g	14 oz
25 g	1 oz	425 g	15 oz
50 g	1 ¾ oz	450 g	1 lb
75 g	2 ¾ oz	500 g	1 lb 2 oz
100 g	3 ½ oz	700 g	1 ½ lb
150 g	5 ½ oz	750 g	1 lb 10 oz
175 g	6 oz	1 kg	2 ¼ lb
200 g	7 oz	1.25 kg	2 lb 12 oz
225 g	8 oz	1.5 kg	3 lb 5 oz
250 g	9 oz	2 kg	4 ½ lb
275 g	9 ¾ oz	2.25 kg	5 lb
300 g	10 ½ oz	2.5 kg	5 ½ lb
350 g	12 oz	3 kg	6 ½ lb

Note: 1 kg is equal to about 2.2 lb.

http://photosimagesvip.com/weight-conversion-table-chart

Temperature Conversion Table

Fahrenheit (°F)	Centigrade (°C)
96.8	36.0
97.7	35.5
98.6	37.0
99.5	37.5
100.4	38.0
101.0	38.3
102.2	39.0
103.1	39.5
104.0	40

Note: To convert °F to °C subtract 32, then multiply by 5/9.
To convert °C to °F multiply by 9/5, then add 32.

Length Conversion Table

Inches	Millimeters	Inches	Millimeters	Inches	Millimeters
1 $\frac{1}{16}$	26.99	3 $\frac{1}{16}$	77.79	5 $\frac{1}{16}$	128.59
1 $\frac{3}{32}$	27.78	3 $\frac{3}{32}$	78.58	5 $\frac{3}{32}$	129.38
1 $\frac{1}{8}$	28.58	3 $\frac{1}{8}$	79.38	5 $\frac{1}{8}$	130.18
1 $\frac{5}{32}$	29.37	3 $\frac{5}{32}$	80.17	5 $\frac{5}{32}$	130.97
1 $\frac{3}{16}$	30.16	3 $\frac{3}{16}$	80.96	5 $\frac{1}{8}$	130.18
1 $\frac{7}{32}$	30.96	3 $\frac{7}{32}$	81.76	5 $\frac{5}{32}$	130.97
1 $\frac{1}{4}$	31.75	3 $\frac{1}{4}$	82.55	5 $\frac{3}{16}$	131.76
1 $\frac{9}{32}$	32.54	3 $\frac{9}{32}$	83.34	5 $\frac{7}{32}$	132.56
1 $\frac{5}{16}$	33.34	3 $\frac{5}{16}$	84.14	5 $\frac{1}{4}$	133.35
1 $\frac{11}{32}$	34.13	3 $\frac{11}{32}$	84.93	5 $\frac{9}{32}$	134.14

(continued)

Length Conversion Table (*continued*)

Inches	Millimeters	Inches	Millimeters	Inches	Millimeters
1 $\frac{3}{8}$	34.93	3 $\frac{3}{8}$	85.73	5 $\frac{5}{16}$	134.94
1 $\frac{13}{32}$	35.72	3 $\frac{13}{32}$	86.52	5 $\frac{11}{32}$	135.73
1 $\frac{7}{16}$	36.51	3 $\frac{7}{16}$	87.31	5 $\frac{3}{8}$	136.53
1 $\frac{15}{32}$	37.31	3 $\frac{15}{32}$	88.11	5 $\frac{13}{32}$	137.32
1 $\frac{1}{2}$	38.10	3 $\frac{1}{2}$	88.90	5 $\frac{7}{16}$	138.11
1 $\frac{17}{32}$	38.89	3 $\frac{17}{32}$	89.69	5 $\frac{15}{32}$	138.91
1 $\frac{9}{16}$	39.69	3 $\frac{9}{16}$	90.49	5 $\frac{1}{2}$	139.70
1 $\frac{19}{32}$	40.48	3 $\frac{19}{32}$	91.28	5 $\frac{17}{32}$	140.49
1 $\frac{5}{8}$	41.28	3 $\frac{5}{8}$	92.08	5 $\frac{9}{16}$	141.29
1 $\frac{21}{32}$	42.07	3 $\frac{21}{32}$	92.87	5 $\frac{19}{32}$	142.08
1 $\frac{11}{16}$	42.86	3 $\frac{11}{16}$	93.66	5 $\frac{5}{8}$	142.88
1 $\frac{23}{32}$	43.66	3 $\frac{23}{32}$	94.46	5 $\frac{21}{32}$	143.67
1 $\frac{3}{4}$	44.45	3 $\frac{3}{4}$	95.25	5 $\frac{11}{16}$	144.66
1 $\frac{25}{32}$	45.24	3 $\frac{25}{32}$	96.04	5 $\frac{23}{32}$	145.26
1 $\frac{13}{16}$	46.04	3 $\frac{13}{16}$	96.84	5 $\frac{3}{4}$	146.05
1 $\frac{27}{32}$	46.83	3 $\frac{27}{32}$	97.63	5 $\frac{25}{32}$	146.84
1 $\frac{7}{8}$	47.63	3 $\frac{7}{8}$	98.43	5 $\frac{13}{16}$	147.64
1 $\frac{29}{32}$	48.42	3 $\frac{29}{32}$	99.22	5 $\frac{27}{32}$	148.43
1 $\frac{15}{16}$	49.21	3 $\frac{15}{16}$	100.01	5 $\frac{7}{8}$	149.23
1 $\frac{31}{32}$	50.01	3 $\frac{31}{32}$	100.81	5 $\frac{29}{32}$	150.02
2	50.80	4	101.60	5 $\frac{15}{16}$	150.81
2 $\frac{1}{32}$	51.59	4 $\frac{1}{32}$	102.39	5 $\frac{31}{32}$	151.61

http://www.sampletemplates.com/business-templates/metric-conversion-chart.html

Appendix C

Drug Classifications

Modified Drug Classification Reference Table From the Children's Hospital Association					
Classification	Examples	Mechanism of Action	Indications	Dosage Considerations	Possible Adverse Effects*
Opioids	Morphine Hydromorphone Codeine Hydrocodone Oxycodone Fentanyl Methadone	Binds to the opioid receptors in the brain and spinal cord during the transmission process	Moderate to severe pain	Titrate to effect (desired analgesia) or intolerable side effects (respiratory depression)	Respiratory depression, nausea, vomiting, constipation, sedation, and urinary retention
Nonopioids	Acetaminophen Aspirin Ibuprofen Naproxen Ketorolac	Inhibits prostaglandin production during the transduction process	Mild to moderate pain, opioidsparing effect, pain secondary to inflammatory conditions	Nonopioids have a "ceiling of analgesia" characteristic, which means that exceeding the recommended mg/kg dose will not provide increased pain relief. Therefore, if the recommended dose does not relieve pain, the clinician should consider adding an opioid.	Dyspepsia, nausea, vomiting, gastrointestinal bleeding, inhibition of platelet aggregation, acute renal failure, and hepatic toxicity

| Local anesthetics | Lidocaine
Bupivacaine
EMLA® | Prevents depolarization and blocks the action during the transduction process | Infiltration of surgical incision or wound for peripheral nerve block

Topical application for numbing the skin prior to needle-stick procedures

Component of epidural infusion | Titrate to effect; exceeding recommended dosing can increase risk of systemic toxicity. | Signs of systemic toxicity include nausea, vomiting, tinnitus, blurred vision, hallucinations, weakness, restlessness, anxiety, dizziness, seizures, bradycardia, palpitations, hypotension, apnea, metallic taste, and cardiac arrest.

Topical agents can cause contact dermatitis, burning, and/or edema. |

(continued)

Classification	Examples	Mechanism of Action	Indications	Dosage Considerations	Possible Adverse Effects*
Anticonvulsants	Gabapentin Carbamazepine Phenytoin Clonazepam Valproic acid Levetiracetam	Primary indication is not analgesia (additional pain management measures need to be taken). The mechanism of anticonvulsants' effect on pain is believed to be prevention of depolarization and blocking the action potential during the transduction process.	Neuropathic pain	Titrate to relief or intolerable side effects	Adverse effects vary with different anticonvulsants and may also be dose dependent (see Chapter 6, "Coanalgesics" for additional information).

| Corticosteroids | Dexamethasone Methylprednisolone Prednisone | Unknown, but may be related to interference with prostaglandin synthesis during the transduction process; shrinkage of tumor mass; tempering of aberrant electrical activity | Neuropathic pain Cancer pain Arthralgia Obstruction pain | A higher dose can be used for acute episodes of severe pain, whereas a lower dose is recommended for chronic, responsive pain. | Associated with administration and withdrawal; risk increases with dose and duration (see Chapter 6, "Coanalgesics" for additional information). |

(continued)

Modified Drug Classification Reference Table From the Children's Hospital Association (continued)					
Classification	Examples	Mechanism of Action	Indications	Dosage Considerations	Possible Adverse Effects*
NMDA receptor antagonist	Ketamine Methadone	Blocks NMDA receptors at the dorsal horn of the spinal cord during the transmission process. May have other analgesic effects	Neuropathic pain Procedural pain Refractory nociceptive pain	Specific to the actual medication	Nausea, vomiting, drowsiness, sedation, and hallucinations
Alpha2-adrenergic agonists	Clonidine	Not established. (See Chapter 6, "Coanalgesics" for additional information.)	Neuropathic pain	Start with low dose and gradually titrate to relief or intolerable adverse effects	Sedation Hypotension Dry mouth

| GABA agonist | Baclofen
Lorazapam
Diazepam | Inhibits transmission of monosynaptic and polysynaptic reflexes at the spinal cord during the modulation process | Neuropathic pain
Possible acute nociceptive pain | Start with low dose and gradually titrate to relief or intolerable adverse effects | Dizziness
Sedation
Nausea
Constipation with coadministration of opiates; may increase the side effects of dizziness and sedation; withdrawal symptom or seizures if stopped abruptly |

GABA, gamma-aminobutyric acid; NMDA, N-methyl-D-aspartate receptor.

*Note that the potency of opioids varies; when switching from one opioid to another, it is important to utilize an equianalgesic table.

Eight Rights of Medication Administration
■ Right patient
■ Right drug
■ Right dose
■ Right route
■ Right time
■ Right documentation
■ Right reason
■ Right response

Source: Bonsall (2012).

Opioids for Neonates

Name of Drug	Use	Dose and Administration	Adverse Effects	Special Considerations
Fentanyl	Analgesia, sedation, and anesthesia	Sedation/analgesia: 0.5–4 mcg/kg per dose IV slow push Infusion rate: 1–5 mcg/kg/hr Anesthesia: 5–50 mcg/kg	Respiratory depression, chest wall rigidity, and urinary retention	Have Naloxone readily available
Methadone	Treatment of opiate withdrawal	Initial dose: 0.05–0.2 mg/kg every 12–24 hr Reduce dose by 10%–20% per week over 4–6 wk	Respiratory depression, ileus and delayed gastric emptying, and QT prolongation	Cardiac assessment and careful weaning
Morphine	Analgesia, sedation, treatment of withdrawal	0.05–0.02 mg/kg IV over at least 5 min Continuous infusion: loading dose of 100–150 mcg/kg over 1 hr followed by 10–20 mcg/kg/hr Treatment of opioid dependence: begin at most recent intravenous (IV) morphine dose; taper 10%–20% per day; oral dose is approximately 3–5 times the IV dose Initial treatment of neonatal narcotic withdrawal: 0.03–0.1 mg/kg per dose orally every 3–4 hr; wean dose 10%–20% every 2/3 days	Respiratory depression, abdominal distention, ileus, and urinary retention	Have Naloxone readily available; protect from light

Adapted from Young and Mangum (2009).

Coanalgesics for Neonates

Name of Drug	Use	Dose and Administration	Adverse Effects	Special Considerations
Acetaminophen	Antipyretic; mild to moderate pain	Oral loading dose: 20–25 mg/kg Maintenance: 12–15 mg/kg Maintenance intervals: Term: every 6 hr Preterm > 32 wk: every 8 hr Preterm < 32 wk: every 12 hr	Liver toxicity with excessive dosing, rash, fever	
NSAIDs	Mild to moderate pain PDA closure	No current recommendations for pain management	Thrombocytopenia, decreased urine output	
EMLA	Topical analgesia	Apply 1–2 g; cover with occlusive dressing for 60–90 min prior to procedure	Blanching, redness, and methemoglobinemia	
Midazolam	Sedation, anesthesia induction, and refractory seizures	IV: 0.05–0.15 mg/kg **over at least 5 min** Repeat every 2–4 hr PRN Oral: 0.25 mg/kg per dose	Respiratory depression and arrest, hypotension	No rapid infusion

Dexme-detomidine	Sedation	Loading dose: 1 mcg/kg Maintenance: 0.5–0.8 mcg/kg		
Phenobarbital	Anticonvulsant	Loading dose: 20 mg/kg, slowly Maintenance: 3–4 mg/kg per day	Respiratory depression	Close management of IV site
Lorazepam	Anticonvulsant	0.05–0.1 mg/kg	Respiratory depression	Dose dependent CNS depression
Thiopental	Sedation	Up to 2mg/kg; max dose 4 mg/kg		
Lidocaine	Dorsal penile block	Less than 37 wk: 0.5 g Greater than 37 wk: 1 g/kg		Allow at least 5 min for effective pain block before procedure begins

CNS, central nervous system; IV, intravenous; NSAIDs, nonsteroidal anti-inflammatory drugs; PDA, patent ductus arteriosis; PRN, as needed or as the situation arises.

Adapted from Young and Magnum (2009).

Index

Printed in the United States
By Bookmasters